T0219637

Genomic Clinical Trials and Predictive Medicine

Genomics is having a major impact on therapeutics development in medicine. This book contains up-to-date information on the use of genomics in the design and analysis of therapeutic clinical trials with a focus on novel approaches that provide a reliable basis for identifying what kinds of patients are likely to benefit from the test treatment. It is oriented to both statisticians and clinical investigators. For clinical investigators, it includes background information on clinical trial design and statistical analysis. For statisticians and others who want to go deeper, it covers state-of-the-art adaptive designs and the development and validation of probabilistic classifiers. The author describes the development and validation of prognostic and predictive biomarkers and their integration into clinical trials that establish their clinical utility for informing treatment decisions for future patients.

Dr. Richard M. Simon is chief of the Biometric Research Branch of the National Cancer Institute, where he is head statistician for the Division of Cancer Treatment and Diagnosis. He is the lead author of the textbook *Design and Analysis of DNA Microarray Experiments* and has more than 450 publications. Dr. Simon has been influential in promoting excellence in clinical trial design and analysis. He has served on the Oncologic Advisory Committee of the U.S. Food and Drug Administration and is a frequent advisor to government, academic, and industry organizations involved with developing improved treatments and diagnostics for patients with cancer. In 1998, Dr. Simon established the Molecular Statistics and Bioinformatics Section of the National Cancer Institute, a multidisciplinary group of scientists developing and applying methods for the application of genomics to cancer therapeutics. He is the architect of BRB-ArrayTools software for the analysis of microarray expression and copy number data.

Practical Guides to Biostatistics and Epidemiology

Series Advisors

Susan Ellenberg, *University of Pennsylvania School of Medicine*
Robert C. Elston, *Case Western Reserve University School of Medicine*
Brian Everitt, *Institute for Psychiatry, King's College London*
Frank Harrell, *Vanderbilt University Medical Center, Tennessee*
Jos W. R. Twisk, *VU University Medical Center, Amsterdam*

This series of short and practical but authoritative books is for biomedical researchers, clinical investigators, public health researchers, epidemiologists, and nonacademic and consulting biostatisticians who work with data from biomedical and epidemiological and genetic studies. Some books explore a modern statistical method and its applications, others may focus on a particular disease or condition and the statistical techniques most commonly used in studying it.

The series is for people who use statistics to answer specific research questions. Books will explain the application of techniques, specifically the use of computational tools, and emphasize the interpretation of results, not the underlying mathematical and statistical theory.

Published in the Series:
Applied Multilevel Analysis, by **Jos W. R. Twisk**
Secondary Data Sources for Public Health, by **Sarah Boslaugh**
Survival Analysis for Epidemiologic and Medical Research, by **Steve Selvin**
Statistical Learning for Biomedical Data, by **James D. Malley**, **Karen G. Malley**, and **Sinisa Pajevic**
Measurement in Medicine, by **Henrica C. W. de Vet**, **Caroline B. Terwee**, **Lidwine B. Mokkink**, and **Dirk L. Knol**

Genomic Clinical Trials and Predictive Medicine

Richard M. Simon

National Cancer Institute

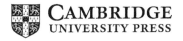

CAMBRIDGE
UNIVERSITY PRESS

CAMBRIDGE
UNIVERSITY PRESS

University Printing House, Cambridge CB2 8BS, United Kingdom

One Liberty Plaza, 20th Floor, New York, NY 10006, USA

477 Williamstown Road, Port Melbourne, VIC 3207, Australia

314-321, 3rd Floor, Plot 3, Splendor Forum, Jasola District Centre, New Delhi - 110025, India

79 Anson Road, #06-04/06, Singapore 079906

Cambridge University Press is part of the University of Cambridge.

It furthers the University's mission by disseminating knowledge in the pursuit of
education, learning and research at the highest international levels of excellence.

www.cambridge.org
Information on this title: www.cambridge.org/9781107401358

First published 2013

A catalogue record for this publication is available from the British Library

Library of Congress Cataloging in Publication data
Simon, Richard M., 1943–
Genomic clinical trials and predictive medicine / Richard M. Simon.
  p. ; cm. – (Practical guides to biostatistics and epidemiology)
Includes bibliographical references and index.
ISBN 978-1-107-00880-9 (hardback) – ISBN 978-1-107-40135-8 (pbk.)
I. Title.   II. Series: Practical guides to biostatistics and epidemiology. [DNLM: 1. Clinical Trials as
Topic – methods.   2. Genomics – methods.   3. Individualized Medicine – methods.
4. Neoplasms – genetics.   5. Research Design.   6. TumorMarkers, Biological – genetics. QU 58.5]
610.72′4–dc23   2012027613

ISBN 978-1-107-00880-9 Hardback
ISBN 978-1-107-40135-8 Paperback

Additional resources for this publication at http://brb.nci.nih.gov.

....

Contents

	Acknowledgments	*page* ix
	Introduction	xi
1	Clinical Trial Basics	1
2	Actionable Prognostic Biomarkers	7
3	Phase II Designs	25
4	Enrichment Designs	35
5	Including Both Test-Positive and Test-Negative Patients	45
6	Adaptive Threshold Design	59
7	Multiple Predictive Biomarkers: Predictive Analysis of Clinical Trials	65
8	Prospective–Retrospective Design	83
	Appendix A. Statistics Background	91
	Appendix B. Prognostic Classifiers Based on High-Dimensional Data	105
	References	129
	Index	139

Acknowledgments

I would like to acknowledge many of the people who directly and indirectly made this book possible: Drs. Robert Wittes and James Doroshow for their friendship and support of my work; my sons Jonathan and Noah Simon for making my life rich and full of love; my past post-doctoral Fellows Drs. Yingdong Zhao, Michael Radmacher, Kevin Dobbin, Abubakar Maitournam, Annette Molinaro, Sudhir Varma, Wenyu Jiang, Jyothi Subramanian, Kyung-In Kim, and Stella Karuri for working with me on much of the material described here; my colleagues Drs. Ed Korn, Larry Rubinstein, Boris Freidlin, and Lisa McShane for freeing me to pursue the study of genomics in cancer therapeutics; and my mother Rose Lander Simon Aach, my sister Florine Simon Bender Marks, and my friend Dr. Joseph Slavin for their love and their courage. Finally, I would like to thank the many clinical and basic scientists and statisticians I have worked with and learned from and all the men and women who dedicate their lives to helping patients with cancer and other debilitating diseases.

Introduction

Genomics is having a major impact on therapeutics development in medicine. In oncology, the impact is particularly profound. Cancer is a set of diseases resulting from DNA alterations, and each tumor is almost unique with regard to the somatic alterations that it harbors. In fact, not only do any two tumors differ with regard to their DNA alterations but each tumor is composed of subclones of cells, and the subclones differ from each other with regard to their mutational spectrum. Although the discovery of these DNA changes provides a rich source of potential molecular targets, the development and evaluation of therapeutics based on re-regulating these targets poses profound challenges, many of which are the topic of this monograph.

Our focus will be heavily on oncology, where the personalization of therapy is primarily based on the tumor DNA genome that has undergone somatic alterations. The material here should be of value, however, in the study of other diseases for which the candidate characteristics for disease personalization are often based on germ line polymorphisms or phenotypic measures of disease heterogeneity.

The randomized clinical trial has been a fundamentally important contribution to medicine. Randomized clinical trials have permitted us to distinguish the minority of new regimens that are effective from the majority of proposed interventions that are ineffective, harmful, and expensive. The history of medicine contains many examples of harmful treatments that persisted for decades based on erroneous expert opinion. Clinical trials attempt to make the opinion of medical authorities evidence based. Of course, we all know that data can be as misleading as authorities, and so clinical trials are rigidly structured to avoid the bias and errors of many data analyses. As a result, however, clinical trials tend to be rather crude tools for answering simple questions. One of the challenges is whether they can be adapted to the more complex questions involved in the personalization of therapeutics, while retaining the high level of reliability in the conclusions that we have come to expect from randomized clinical trials.

In addition to addressing the development of therapeutics, this monograph is about the development and evaluation of diagnostic tests for enabling the right drug to be used for the right patient. There is currently an enormous amount of confusion, hype, and misinformation published about personalized medicine biomarkers.

Although this monograph is not a primer on clinical trials, I have included an introductory chapter that may serve as a useful introduction for some readers and be skipped by others. I include an appendix that covers the basic statistical background needed for the material in this text for nonstatistical readers. The second chapter addresses biomarkers, prognostic classifiers, and the evaluation of diagnostic tests. The subsequent chapters describe designs and analysis strategies for the use of genomics in prospective clinical trials. Chapter 7 also includes material on the development and validation of multivariate predictive classifiers for identifying patients whose prognosis is better on a specified treatment than a control. Most of the analysis methods described in Chapter 7 and Appendix B are available in the BRB-ArrayTools software (Simon et al. 2007) available at http://brb.nci.nih.gov. Chapter 8 describes the prospective–retrospective approach to evaluate the medical utility of prognostic and predictive biomarkers based on previously conducted clinical trials. I also include an appendix on the development and validation of prognostic biomarkers using high-dimensional data such as gene expression profiles.

The target audience of the monograph includes statisticians, clinical investigators, and translational scientists. The focus is on new approaches to the design of clinical trials with prospectively specified analysis plans that provide a reliable basis for identifying what kinds of patients are likely to benefit from the test treatment. The focus is not on statistically complicated model-based analyses. There is abundant literature on post hoc analysis of clinical trials using complex statistical models. The problem is that the post hoc approach does not result in the kind of reliable conclusion that we expect from phase III clinical trials, so those analyses are considered exploratory and hypothesis generating for future trials. Here we emphasize designing a clinical trial and prespecifying an analysis plan so that one obtains information about whether the test treatment has any benefit and, if so, whether a reliable classifier that characterizes the patients who are most likely to benefit from the test treatment can be obtained.

The book includes novel designs and novel approaches that have been developed in the past several years. Web-based programs are available at http://brb.nci.nih.gov for utilizing some of the designs. For some of the designs discussed, sufficient time has not passed for there to be published examples. These designs are currently of considerable interest in oncology drug development. I hope that the monograph contains accessible material of importance for readers of diverse backgrounds and that it can help in our efforts to develop more effective treatments for debilitating diseases.

Clinical Trial Basics

We will present here a brief review of some of the key aspects of therapeutic clinical trials. In oncology, clinical trials are often categorized into phase I, phase II, and phase III trials. Phase I trials are conducted to determine the maximum dose at which a new drug can be delivered in a defined schedule of administration before dose-limiting toxicity occurs. Phase I trials may also evaluate the pharmacokinetics of the drug administration schedule and the pharmacodynamics of whether the drug inhibits its molecular target. Phase II trials are conducted to identify whether a new drug has antitumor activity when administered as a single agent or whether it contributes to the antitumor activity of other drugs. Phase II trials are traditionally conducted in patients with a particular histologic diagnosis and stage of disease. Traditionally, phase II trials of chemotherapeutic drugs are conducted in a wide range of types of cancer to screen for activity sufficiently great to warrant a phase III trial. With the advent of molecularly targeted drugs, an increasingly important objective of phase II trials is to develop a pretreatment biological measurement, that is, a *biomarker*, that can be used to identify the patients whose tumors are the most likely to benefit from the drug. Phase II trials do not generally establish the medical utility of a new drug or new regimen; that is the role of phase III trials. Phase II trials generally use an intermediate end-point that reflects antitumor activity but has not been established as a valid measure of patient benefit. The phase II trials determine whether the new drug is sufficiently promising to evaluate in a larger phase III trial and, if so, what the target population should be and how the new drug should be administered.

Phase III clinical trials are generally large studies in which patients who satisfy predefined eligibility criteria are randomized to receive either the new regimen or a control regimen, usually representing a standard of care. There is generally a primary end-point, or measure of effectiveness, that represents a direct measure of patient benefit such as survival or survival without evidence of disease. The end-point is the same for both the new treatment being evaluated and the control, and great care is taken to plan follow-up surveillance of the patients so that the end-point can be evaluated equivalently for the two treatment arms. The plans for accruing, evaluating, and treating patients, collecting data, and performing data analyses are rigorously specified in a written protocol so that a medically meaningful and statistically reliable assessment of a well-defined population of patients, carefully staged and homogeneously treated, can result (Simon, 2011, 828; Piantadosi, 2005; Crowley and Hoering, 2012).

Statistically, most phase III clinical trials have been structured to test a single null hypothesis that the distribution of outcomes for the new treatment is equivalent to that of the control with regard to the primary end-point overall for all randomized patients. The *intention to treat principle* is observed in the analysis; that is, all eligible randomized patients are included in the primary null hypothesis test regardless of whether or not they received their assigned treatment as defined in the protocol. The intention to treat principle is counterintuitive to many physicians. Why retain a patient in the treatment arm to which he or she was randomized if he or she did not receive that treatment or if the treatment wasn't administered in the way it was intended (Piantadosi, 2005, 829; Green, Benedetti, & Crowley, 2003, 322)? The purpose of the intention to treat principle is to ensure that the prognostic comparability created by randomization is not destroyed by the exclusion of prognostically unfavorable patients from one arm more than the other. By comparing the outcomes of the patients as randomized, one avoids false positive findings resulting from biased exclusions. The intention to treat principle may increase the false negative rate (i.e., decrease the statistical power) of the trial. In oncology clinical trials, it is common to exclude patients who were not actually eligible for the clinical trial but not to exclude any eligible randomized patients. If there are numerous major treatment violations for eligible randomized patients, the credibility of the trial may be compromised to an extent that cannot be rescued by statistical analysis.

At the time of the final analysis, a single null hypothesis of no average treatment effect is tested by computing a test statistic that summarizes a difference in average outcomes between the group randomized to the new treatment and the control group. With survival or disease-free survival data, a log-rank statistic is used. The probability of obtaining a value of the test statistic as great as that computed from the data is calculated under the assumption that the null hypothesis is true. That probability is called the *p value* or the statistical significance level. A one-sided *p* value is the probability, under the null hypothesis, of obtaining a value of the test statistic as great as that computed from the data and in the direction favoring the new treatment. A two-sided *p* value is the probability under the null hypothesis of obtaining a value of the test statistic as great in absolute value as that computed from the data in either direction. Although most phase III clinical trials compare a new treatment to a control, results are usually only reported as statistically significant if the two-sided *p* value is less than 0.05. This assures that only 2.5% of phase III clinical trials will be reported as finding new treatments statistically significantly better than control groups.

The size and duration of phase III clinical trials are usually planned so that if the true degree of benefit of the new treatment versus control is of a prespecified magnitude Δ, then the probability of obtaining a statistically significant result will be large, usually 80% or 90%. The Δ value is called the *treatment effect* to be detected and the 80% or 90% is called the *statistical power*. The power is a function of the Δ value, the number of patients, and the follow-up time. For survival or disease-free survival data, a commonly used formula is

$$E_{\text{tot}} = 4\frac{\left(k_{1-\alpha} + k_{1-\beta}\right)^2}{\Delta^2}. \tag{1.1}$$

In formula (1.1), E_{tot} denotes the total number of events to be detected at the time of the final analysis. If the primary end-point is survival, then an event is death. If the primary end-point is disease-free survival, then an event is the earlier of disease recurrence or death. The constants $k_{1-\alpha}$ and $k_{1-\beta}$ in the numerator of (1.1) are percentiles of the standard normal distribution, α is the desired one-sided significance level of the test (usually 0.025), and $1 - \beta$ is the desired statistical power. For

$\alpha = 0.025$ and $1 - \beta = 0.80, k_{1-0.025} = 1.96$ and $k_{0.80} = 0.84$. For 90% power, the latter constant becomes 1.28. This approach to sample size planning is based on the assumption of proportional hazards for survival or disease-free survival data. Variable Δ represents the natural logarithm of the ratio of the hazard of death for a patient on the new treatment relative to the hazard of death for a patient on the control. With a proportional hazards model, the ratio of hazard of death at time t for a patient on the new treatment relative to a patient on control is the same for all times t. Phase III clinical trials are often planned to detect reductions in the hazard by 25–40%. A 33% reduction in hazard corresponds to $\Delta = \log(0.67) = -0.40$.

For proportional hazards models, the statistical power is determined by the number of events at the time of final analysis rather than by the number of patients. The number of total events at any time is, however, a function of both the number of patients and the follow-up time relative to the survival distributions. For such survival studies, the timing of the final analysis is best indicated in terms of number of events, not absolute calendar time.

A very important feature of (1.1) is that the required number of events is proportional to the reciprocal of the square of the size of the treatment effect to be detected, Δ. This is generally true, not just for proportional hazard models, nor just for survival data. A small increase in the size of the treatment effect to be detected results in a large decrease in the required size of the study. This provides an important motivation for the search for predictive biomarkers that will enable the eligibility criteria to be restricted to patients for whom the treatment effect is likely to be large. Use of even an imperfect predictive biomarker can result in a large reduction in the required size of the study. The size of the treatment effect can be increased either by excluding patients unlikely to do well on the new treatment or by excluding patients who do very well on the control.

The process of planning the size of a clinical trial sometimes ignores the interim analyses that will be conducted. The statistical features of the interim analyses must, however, be detailed in the protocol. The type I error of the clinical trial is the probability that the null hypothesis is falsely rejected at any analysis, interim or final. Consequently, the threshold significance levels for declaring statistical significance at individual interim and final levels must be reduced below 0.05 if the total type I error is to be limited to 0.05 (Pocock, 1982, 425; Fleming, 1989, 303; Jennison & Turnbull, 1999, 344). One conservative approach would be to have each threshold be $0.05/(I + 1)$, where I is the number of interim analyses. This approach is rarely used in oncology trials. A more common approach is to use a threshold of 0.045 for the final analysis and to use very extreme thresholds like 0.001 for the interim analyses (Haybittle, 1971, 332; O'Brien & Fleming, 1979, 406). This has little effect on the statistical power computed ignoring the interim analyses but provides relatively little likelihood of stopping early. For large multicenter clinical trials, the latter philosophy is often desired because the interim analyses are conducted with incompletely quality-controlled data.

For most phase III clinical trials, the results of the interim analyses are kept blinded to investigators entering patients in the trial and are reviewed by a data safety monitoring committee consisting of individuals with no conflict of interest and who are not entering patients in the trial (Smith et al., 1997, 504; Ellenberg, Fleming, & DeMets, 2002, 292). The purpose of the data monitoring committee is to maintain the equipoise of physicians who enter patients in the clinical trial while ensuring that the patients are protected.

If the null hypothesis is rejected at an interim or final analysis, then generally, the new treatment is recommended for all future patients who satisfy the eligibility criteria for the study. If the null hypothesis is not rejected, then the new treatment is not recommended for regulatory approval or future use outside clinical trials. Although subset analyses are often performed, those results are generally viewed skeptically by statisticians (Fleming, 1995, 300; Pocock et al., 2002, 426). Some statisticians use the rule of thumb of not believing the subset analysis unless the primary overall null hypothesis is rejected. This reflects the importance to statisticians of protecting the overall type I error for the study. It also reflects an implicit prior belief that new treatments usually do not work, so it is better to believe that some subsets do not benefit when the overall null hypothesis is rejected than it is to believe that some subsets do benefit when the overall null hypothesis is not rejected. This focus on the overall analysis was reflective of an era of blockbuster drugs for homogeneous diseases. This approach has protected physicians from false positive results based on post-hoc subset analyses with ineffective drugs. The approach has led to overtreatment of many patients based on statistically significant but small average treatment effects in large clinical trials with broad eligibility criteria. For study of molecularly heterogeneous diseases in which treatment effects are expected to vary among patients, the methods described in this monograph for development of companion diagnostics for refining therapeutic decision making take on increased importance.

2

Actionable Prognostic Biomarkers

Biological measurements used to inform treatment selection are sometimes called biomarkers, but the term invites misinterpretation. Many people think of biomarkers as measures of disease activity, increasing as the disease progresses and decreasing as the disease responds. Such disease biomarkers would have considerable utility as surrogate end-points for clinical trials. Regulatory agencies are, of course, very concerned about accepting a surrogate end-point as a basis for drug approval. Although biomarkers are commonly used as end-points in phase I and phase II clinical trials to establish that a drug inhibits its target or has antidisease activity and for selecting among doses, very stringent criteria have been established for validating surrogate end-points for use in phase III clinical trials. It is generally very difficult to establish that a biological measurement is a valid "disease biomarker." Our focus here is on prognostic and predictive baseline biomarkers, not on surrogate end-points.

Prognostic markers are pretreatment measurements that provide information about long-term outcome for patients who are either untreated or receive standard treatment. Prognostic markers often reflect a combination of intrinsic disease factors and sensitivity to standard therapy. Predictive biomarkers identify patients who are likely or unlikely to benefit from a specific treatment. For example, HER2 amplification is a predictive biomarker for benefit from trastuzumab. A predictive biomarker may be used to identify patients who are poor candidates for a particular drug; for example, colorectal cancer patients whose tumors have KRAS mutations are poor candidates for treatment with anti-EGFR monoclonal antibodies. Most of the following chapters address the development and validation of predictive biomarkers for guiding the use of a new treatment. In this chapter, however, we discuss the development and validation of prognostic biomarkers that have medical utility for informing treatment decisions.

Although many diseases feature a large literature of prognostic factor studies, relatively few such tests are recommended by professional societies, reimbursed by payers, or widely ordered by practicing physicians (Pusztai, 2004, 641). Published studies are rarely planned with an intended use in mind. The cases included represent a convenience sample of patients for whom preserved tissue is available. These patients are often heterogeneous with regard to treatment, staging procedures used, and extent of disease. The prognostic factors identified are often not helpful in making treatment decisions. The studies are often motivated by the hope of better understanding the pathogenesis of the disease rather than by plans for developing a test with medical utility.

In discussing medical tests, three types of validity can be distinguished: *analytical validity, clinical validity*, and *medical utility* (Simon, Paik, & Hayes, 2009, 684). Analytical validity originally meant that the assay provides an accurate measurement of the quantity that it claims to measure. In some cases, however, there is no gold-standard measurement on which to base the comparison. In such cases, analytical validity is taken to mean that the measurement is reproducible and robust over time, within and between laboratories (Cronin et al., 2007, 806).

Clinical validity means that the test result correlates well with some clinical end-point. Most prognostic factor publications demonstrate some form of clinical validity but not analytical validity or medical utility. Medical utility means that the test result is actionable in a way that results in patient benefit. The action that a test result can inform is often treatment selection. If the test tells something about the patient's disease but there is nothing one can do with that knowledge, then there is no medical utility. In some cases, the patient might want to have that increased knowledge of his or her prognosis, but few payers reimburse for prognostic measurements that are not medically indicated. If the knowledge is actionable but could have been obtained from standard prognostic factors, then there is no incremental medical utility.

How can a new prognostic marker have medical utility? When the standard of care (SOC) is intensive therapy, this can be accomplished by identifying patients who have such good prognosis with conservative treatment that they may choose to forgo more intensive therapy. For example, the Oncotype DX recurrence score was developed for women with newly diagnosed breast cancer that expressed hormonal receptors and had not apparently disseminated to the lymph nodes or beyond (Paik et al., 2004, 411). At the time of development, the SOC for such women was treatment with hormonal therapy and cytotoxic chemotherapy. The test was developed to identify which breast cancer patients had such good prognoses on hormonal therapy alone that they could opt to forgo chemotherapy. The action involved was withholding chemotherapy, and the benefit to the patient was having an excellent outcome while avoiding the toxicity of chemotherapy.

Developing Oncotype DX as a prognostic marker that would inform treatment decisions required studying patients whose tumors expressed hormonal receptors and had not disseminated to lymph nodes or beyond and who received hormonal therapy as their only systemic treatment. The intended use of the test determined both the selection of patients and the analysis of the study performed for developing the test. Such focused development is unusual and is the primary reason why prognostic markers with medical utility are so unusual.

The analysis and interpretation of the Oncotype DX prognostic study was also unusual. Most prognostic factor studies are analyzed as statistical exercises in significance testing and reporting hazard ratios. Such methods are mostly irrelevant for identifying medical utility, where the key issue is whether the marker identifies a subset of patients who have such excellent prognoses on conservative treatment that they are unlikely to benefit to a meaningful degree from higher-intensity regimens. A more appropriate analysis would simply involve computing the relationship of biomarker value to prognosis with confidence limits. For example, suppose that the marker identifies a subset of patients with an apparent cure rate of more than 95%. Because their outcome on low-intensity treatment is so good, they cannot benefit much, in absolute terms, from higher-intensity treatment. A reduction in hazard of failure of 30%, which is substantial for cancer

treatments, would provide an increase in the cure rate of only 5% ×
30%, or 1.5% (from 95% to 96.5%), in absolute terms, and this may
not be worth the side effects of chemotherapy for many patients. If,
however, the cure rate for the good-prognosis group were only 85%,
then the potential benefit of chemotherapy might be 15% × 30%, or
4.5% (from 85% to 89.5%), in absolute terms, and the prognostic marker
would have less certain utility for informing a decision to withhold more
intensive treatment, particularly when uncertainty in the estimate of the
cure rate is taken into account.

In discussing prognostic markers, treatment is often ignored. However, for developing a prognostic marker with medical utility, treatment
is of fundamental importance. Utility for withholding intensive therapy
can only be established if two conditions prevail: (1) the SOC for the
target population is intensive treatment and (2) the prognostic analysis
is based on patients who did not receive the intensive treatment. These
two conditions prevailed in the development of Oncotype DX. At the
time of development, the SOC for most stage I breast cancer patients
with hormone-receptor-positive tumors was hormonal treatment plus
chemotherapy, but the development was based on data from a clinical trial performed years earlier, when the SOC was hormonal therapy
alone. For examples of much less effective or actionable prognostic classifiers, see the review by Subramanian and Simon (2010, 719–720) of
prognostic gene expression signatures for early lung cancer.

The Oncotype DX recurrence score is a weighted average of the expression levels of 21 genes. The MammaPrint score is a classifier based on the
expression levels of 70 genes (van-de-Vijver et al., 2002, 103; van't-Veer
et al., 2002, 90). We include such composite tests as prognostic markers
because the manner in which a marker is used in a validation clinical
trial is independent of whether it is based on a single measurement
or a summary of multiple measurements. For composite markers like
Oncotype DX and MammaPrint, however, it is essential that the way
the multiple measurements are combined is completely specified, that
is, "locked down." It is not enough just to specify the genes involved;
the weighting factors used in combining the genes and the cut points, if
any, used for treatment decisions must also be specified. Oncotype DX is
based on a weighted average of 21 genes, and so the way those expression

levels are normalized and the weights used must be completely specified. MammaPrint is a "nearest centroid" classifier, and so not only the 70 genes involved but also the centroids of each of those 70 genes in each class must be specified. Oncotype DX provides a continuous prognostic score. MammaPrint classifies patients into good, intermediate, or poor prognosis classes based on the expression level of 70 genes.

A fundamental principle for the validation of the medical utility of a biomarker of any kind is that validation means "fitness for intended use." Thus, the intended use must be specified before one can think properly about what form the validation study should take. With respect to classifiers or scores such as Oncotype DX and MammaPrint, which combine the expression levels of multiple genes in a predefined manner, it is only the combined classifier or score that should be validated, not the individual gene expression measurements. Only the combined classifier or score is used, and so only it needs to be validated as fit for the intended use.

2.1 Design and Analysis of Developmental Studies of Prognostic Classifiers

Developmental studies are generally retrospective studies in which numerous candidate prognostic markers are evaluated. There is, of course, a large body of literature using regression modeling for such applications, but a new body of literature has emerged for developing such models when the number of candidate variables is larger than the number of samples. The development of prognostic models in such settings is reviewed in Appendix B.

As we have already indicated, a key to the design of a meaningful developmental study is specification of the intended use of the prognostic marker to be developed. Cases should be selected for the developmental study based on the intended use. Often this means identifying a target population of patients for whom the current SOC is intensive treatment and for whom you hope to identify a subset with such good prognosis on lower-intensity treatment that the current SOC can be withheld. The developmental study would consist of prognostic modeling of patients in the target population who received low-intensity treatment.

2.1.1 Sample Size Planning

There is substantial literature on sample size planning for finding genes whose expression is correlated with outcome. Finding such genes is not the same, however, as developing a model containing multiple genes that can be used to predict outcome on the low-intensity treatment. Gene finding is only one component of developing a prognostic model. Simon et al. (2002, 154) applied a method previously developed by Hsieh and Lavori (2000) to plan sample size for detecting genes whose expression levels are associated with survival outcome in proportional hazards models. The total number of events required for a gene is given by

$$D = \frac{\left(k_{\alpha/2} + k_\beta\right)^2}{(\tau \ln(\delta))^2} \qquad (2.1)$$

where α and β denote the two-sided type I error and type II error levels, respectively, τ denotes the standard deviation of the log2 gene expression measurement over the samples, and δ denotes the hazard ratio associated with a one-unit change in the log2 expression measurement for the gene. A one-unit change in the log2 expression measurement corresponds to a twofold change in the expression measurement. Because many genes will be tested for association with survival, to control the number of false positives (i.e., "false discoveries"), the threshold significance level α should be made much more stringent than for conventional problems. In testing, an α of 0.001 results in one false discovery per 1,000 null genes tested if the genes are independent. Because genes work in pathways and networks and are not independent, planning sample size using an α of 0.001 is often reasonable. If the proportion of genes that are nonnull is γ and expression values for the G genes tested are independent, then the expected number of false discoveries is $\alpha(1 - \gamma)G$, and the expected number of true discoveries is $(1 - \beta)\gamma G$, so the expected false discovery rate (FDR) can be approximated by

$$\text{FDR} \approx \left\{1 + \frac{\gamma(1 - \beta)}{\alpha(1 - \gamma)}\right\}^{-1}. \qquad (2.2)$$

If $\gamma = 0.1$ (i.e., 10% of the genes are differentially expressed) and $\beta = 0.05$ (i.e., 95% power for detecting each differentially expressed gene), then the FDR is approximately 0.9% for $\alpha = 0.001$ and approximately

4.5% for $\alpha = 0.005$. If $\gamma = 0.05$ and $\beta = 0.05$, then the FDR is approximately 1.8% for $\alpha = 0.001$ and approximately 8.6% for $\alpha = 0.005$. Increasing β to 0.10 has little effect on the FDR but reduces the power for detecting genes associated with survival outcome.

Using expression (2.1) with $\alpha = 0.005$, $\beta = 0.05$, $\delta = 2$, and $\tau = 1$ gives a D of approximately 42 events required. Variables $\delta = 2$ and $\tau = 1$ correspond to a doubling of hazard for a change in log expression level corresponding to 1 standard deviation.

Dobbin and Simon also addressed the problem of sample size planning for developing a classification model for distinguishing two classes, for example, those with good outcome versus those with poor outcome (Dobbin & Simon, 2007, 281; Dobbin, Zhao, & Simon, 2008, 559). They formulated the problem as determining the sample size so that the expected true classification error is no greater than a tolerance ε greater than the classification error for the model that could be built with infinite sample size. Although their results have not been extended for time-to-event data, they can be used heuristically by interpreting the required number of cases as the number of required events.

2.1.2 Clinical Validation

The results in the previous section provide guidelines for planning the number of cases needed for a training set for developing a prognostic model with high-dimensional data. Developmental studies should, however, provide an unbiased estimate of the relation of model-estimated prognosis to outcome. Traditionally in statistics, the same data are used for developing a model and for evaluating the goodness of fit of the model. This works adequately when the number of cases is large relative to the number of candidate variables. It gives misleading results, however, when the number of candidate variables (p) is commensurate with or greater than the number of cases (n). The number of candidate variables is what matters, not the number of variables in the resulting model. If you select the single variable from 1,000 that provides the best apparent fit to a model when there are 100 cases, the resulting fit will be highly optimistically biased.

Subramanian and Simon (2010, 719) demonstrated the large bias that results when estimating the prognostic effect of a survival prognosis model using the same cases as those used for developing the model.

They simulated survival times and expression data for 1,000 genes. The survival times were simulated completely independently of all the gene expression measurements. For each simulated data set, they fit a prognostic proportional hazards model based on the 10 genes with the largest apparent correlation with survival in the data set. They then used that fitted model to classify the same patients according to whether they were predicted to have survival greater than or less than the median for the group. This is not really prediction because the prediction is for the same cases whose survival and gene expression data were used for selecting the best apparent genes for inclusion in the model and for fitting the model. Figure 2.1 (left) shows the Kaplan–Meier survival curves for the cases predicted as having a low risk and a high risk of death. The curves are widely separated in all 10 simulated data sets. Subramanian and Simon then tested the actual predictive ability of these 10 models. They generated gene expression values and survivals for an independent data set using the same independence model used to generate the 10 training sets. The fitted models were then used to classify the patients in the independent data sets as having a good or poor prognosis. The model was not refit to the new data; rather, the model developed on the original data set was used to classify the new patients. Those results are shown in Figure 2.1 (right). In all 10 samples, the models that appeared so impressive when improperly evaluated on the training sets were seen to be worthless when properly evaluated on independent data.

When one has a single data set both for developing and evaluating a prognostic model, two general approaches will avoid the extreme bias shown in Figure 2.1: the *split-sample approach* and the *resampling approach*. The split-sample approach partitions the cases into two components: a training set and a testing or validation set. A single completely specified prognostic model is developed on the training set. This may be a survival classification model that classifies patients into survival risk groups, or it may be a model that provides a continuous prognostic score. The single fully specified model developed on the training set is simply applied to the cases in the validation set. No adjustment of the model for the validation set is permitted. For a survival risk classification model, the validation-set patients are classified into risk groups, and Kaplan–Meier survival curves for the validation-set risk groups are then computed. For models giving a continuous prognostic score, the score is computed for patients in the validation set, those patients are separated into risk groups based on the ranks of their prognostic scores, and the Kaplan–Meier survival curves for these validation-set risk groups are computed. The validation set should not be used in any way in the process of model development. Preferably, the validation-set cases should not even be used for gene filtering or for normalization because the purpose of the exercise is to emulate the process of predicting for a future case, and future samples cannot be used for such purposes. The most frequent error made is to use the full data set for selecting genes and then developing a model on the training set using the selected genes. This produces highly biased results. A second common error is to develop multiple models using the training data and to use the accuracy of the models on the validation set to select among the models developed on the training set. This sometimes takes the form of developing a set of models on the training set, one for each value of a tuning parameter, and then using the validation set to optimize the value of the tuning parameter. This approach also results in bias. A single fully specified model should be developed on the training set before the validation set data are used. If there are tuning parameters to be optimized or different kinds of classification models to be evaluated, then they should be optimized and evaluated using only the training data (Varma & Simon, 2006, 531). In some split-sample approaches, the data are partitioned into three components; the training set is used to select genes and the model form, an intermediate calibration set is used to fit the specified model, and finally, the validation set is used to evaluate the single completely specified model developed on the training and calibration sets.

Generally, the primary measure of model performance to be evaluated on the validation set is whether the model identifies patients with such good prognosis on low-intensity treatment that they do not require a higher-intensity regimen. Unfortunately, the analyses usually performed are not informative with regard to an intended use of the model. Whether the model is statistically significantly prognostic or the size of the hazard ratio between risk groups is not directly relevant. In fact, hazard ratios can be misleading because very large hazard ratios are needed before models are usefully prognostic (Pepe, 2004, 682).

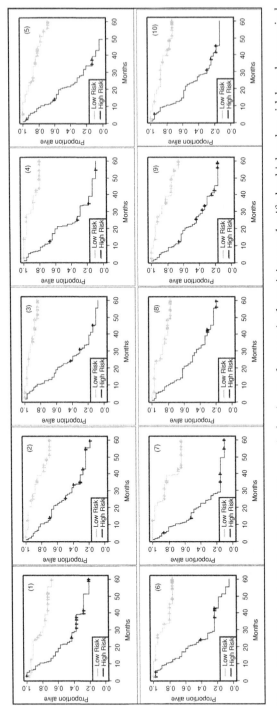

Figure 2.1. (left) Resubstitution Kaplan–Meier survival estimates for cases in the training set classified as high or low risk based on survival risk models developed in the same training set. The training set data were simulated from a model in which none of the variables used for modeling were actually prognostic for survival. Each simulation is numbered. (right) Kaplan–Meier survival estimates for cases in independent test sets classified as high or low risk using the models developed in the corresponding training sets shown in the left panel. Data for the independent test sets were simulated from the same model used for simulating data for the training sets; none of the variables used for modeling was prognostic for survival.

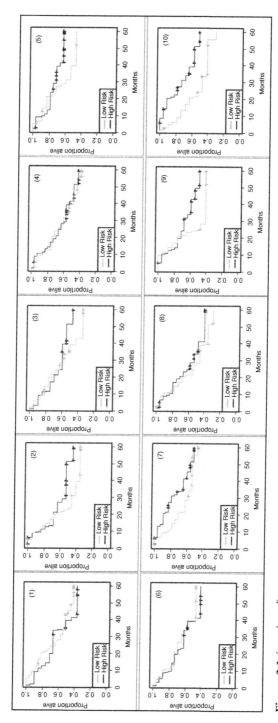

Figure 2.1 (*continued*)

17

Radmacher, McShane, and Simon (2002, 86) discuss planning the size of the validation set when using the split-sample approach. Dobbin and Simon (2011, 835) discuss how to optimally partition an existing data set into a training set and a validation set. The cross-validation of prognostic classifiers for $p > n$ settings is described in detail in Appendix B. The cross-validated Kaplan–Meier curves for the 10 simulated data sets shown in Figure 2.1 (left) are shown in Figure 2.2. Here, we briefly outline the philosophy of the cross-validation approach. When a data set D is partitioned into a training set T and a validation set V, a prognostic classifier is built using the training data. Let $C(;T)$ denote this classifier. For any vector of prognostic variable $\underline{x}$, the classifier $C(\underline{x};T)$ equals 0 or 1 corresponding to the predicted class of the case. The split-sample method uses the validation set V to provide an estimate of the misclassification error rate of the classifier $C(;T)$. If the full data set D is very large, then the training set T will be adequate for development of a classifier and the validation set V will be adequate for evaluating the classifier. In many applications, however, the full data set D is not that large. Consequently, the classifier that can be developed on a training set T may be substantially inferior to the classifier that could be developed on the full data set and the validation set V may be too small to adequately evaluate the classifier developed on T. In these circumstances, resampling or cross-validation (a particular type of resampling) is recommended over the split-sample approach.

With the cross-validation approach, a classifier $C(;D)$ is developed using the full data set D. To estimate the misclassification error rate for future use of $C(;D)$, one cannot simply classify the patients in D using $C(;D)$ and count the errors. This resubstitution estimate of the error is known to be very biased. Instead, the resampling approach uses a different estimate. Let $MER(D)$ denote the misclassification error rate of the classifier $C(;D)$. If one views the data set D as a sample of data sets that could have been obtained to develop the classifier, then $MER(D)$ can be viewed as a random variable with mean $\mu = E_D(MER(D))$, where the right-hand side denotes the expected value of the misclassification error rate with regard to sampling different data sets D. Resampling methods provide an estimate of μ and use that as an estimate of $MER(D)$. The

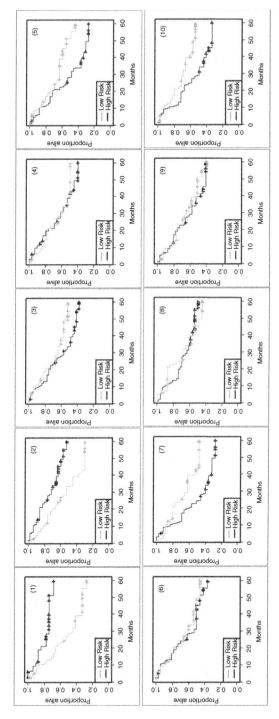

Figure 2.2. Cross-validated Kaplan–Meier survival estimates for the training sets shown in Figure 2.1 (left).

mean μ is estimated by resampling data sets D' without replacement from the original data set D. For each resampled data set D', $MER(D')$ is estimated by evaluating $C(;D')$ on the complement set D-D'. Molinaro et al. (2005, 396) evaluated a variety of different forms of the resampling approach and compared them to the simple split-sample approach for binary classification problems. They found that for small data sets, leave-one-out cross-validation often provided the estimate of $MER(D)$ having the smallest mean-squared error. For larger data sets, fivefold or tenfold cross-validation is often more effective than leave-one-out cross-validation or split sample. For details, see Appendix B.

2.2 Design of Validation Studies of Prognostic Classifiers

A validation study of a prognostic classifier differs from a developmental study in that in the former, the prognostic classifier is determined in advance. The validation study should ideally emulate the tissue-handling and assay performance procedures that would be encountered in clinical practice. This may contrast with the developmental study, in which a nonanalytically validated assay performed retrospectively under research conditions is employed. The validation study should be clearly focused on medical utility, that is, whether the classifier can be used to inform treatment decisions in a manner that results in patient benefit. *Patient benefit* generally means either improved outcome or equivalent outcome with less invasive treatment. An excellent discussions of the evaluation of diagnostic and prognostic biomarkers is given by Pepe et al. (2008).

The most direct design for evaluating medical utility of a classifier is one in which patients are randomized either to receive the SOC or to receive treatment determined or informed by the classifier. This design, illustrated in Figure 2.3, is often called the *marker strategy design*. With a prognostic classifier, the SOC may be an intensive treatment such as chemotherapy following surgery, radiation, and hormonal therapy for women with stage I hormone-receptor-positive breast cancer. With this design, the patients randomized to SOC often do not have the test performed. The patients randomized to the experimental arm would have the test performed, and if the classifier were to indicate that the patient

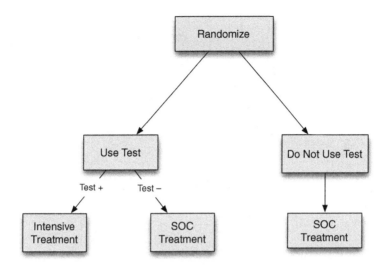

Figure 2.3. Marker strategy design. Patients are randomized to be tested or not. Patients not tested receive standard-of-care treatment. Patients tested receive the treatment informed by the test. This is usually a very inefficient design that requires an excessively large sample size because many patients will receive the same treatment regardless of the randomization.

has good prognosis without chemotherapy, then intensive treatment would be withheld; otherwise, the SOC would be administered.

The marker strategy design is, however, a very inefficient means of evaluating the classifier because many patients will receive the same treatment regardless of whether they are randomized to be tested (Simon, Paik, & Hayes, 2009, 684; Freidlin, McShane, & Korn, 2010, 723). This results in very poor statistical power for detecting whether withholding chemotherapy for patients predicted to have good prognosis is detrimental. It is not valid to compare outcomes for those patients in the experimental arm who had chemotherapy withheld to outcomes for all patients in the control arm. Patients in the experimental arm who had chemotherapy withheld cannot be compared to patients in the control arm who would have had chemotherapy withheld had they been in the other arm because the test is not performed for patients in the control arm.

A better alternative is to use the modified marker strategy design shown in Figure 2.4, in which all patients are tested before randomization, and the only patients randomized are those for whom the marker

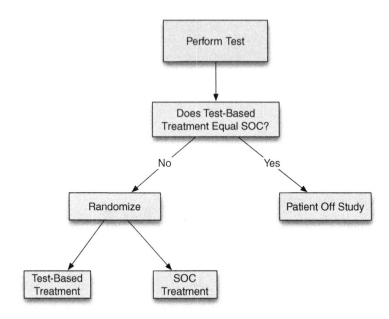

Figure 2.4. Modified marker strategy design. All patients are tested before randomization. Only patients for whom the test informed treatment is different from the standard-of-care treatment are randomized.

determined that treatment differs from the SOC. This design provides much greater power for evaluating the medical utility of the classifier. This is the design used for the MINDACT clinical trial that is testing the medical utility of the MammaPrint prognostic signature for women with stage I, hormone-receptor-positive breast cancer (Bogaerts et al., 2006, 619).

The Oncotype DX recurrence score was originally developed for stage I breast cancer patients with hormone-receptor-positive tumors. The TailoRx clinical trial is a prospective trial to evaluate the Oncotype DX recurrence score (Sparano & Paik, 2008, 620). In this trial, the test is performed for all eligible women. Women predicted to have excellent prognosis without chemotherapy are not randomized, however; they all have chemotherapy withheld. The test will be considered to have utility if the outcome for such patients without chemotherapy is as good as predicted. The philosophy is that if their outcomes are that good, then the benefit of chemotherapy cannot be great enough in absolute terms to be worthwhile, and consequently, a SOC control group for these good-prognosis patients is not needed. Although the MINDACT trial randomizes patients predicted to have very good prognosis without chemotherapy to either SOC chemotherapy or having chemotherapy withheld, the analysis plan and the sample size planning are for a nonrandomized comparison, as in TailoRx.

3

Phase II Designs

The purpose of a phase II clinical trial of a treatment regimen is generally to determine whether the regimen is sufficiently promising to warrant a phase III evaluation and to optimize the regimen and the target population for use in the phase III trial. The objective of optimizing the target population takes on great importance in developing molecularly targeted treatments for biologically heterogeneous diseases. Molecularly targeted treatments often aim to treat the underlying disease mechanism, not the secondary symptoms. Such treatments are generally not expected to be broadly effective for biologically heterogeneous diseases. The phase II studies should evaluate the candidate predictive biomarkers for the one that identifies the best candidates for the new treatment.

For oncology drugs that are specific for a known molecular target, the predictive biomarker candidates have often been measures of overexpression of the target protein in the tumor cells or mutation or amplification of the associated gene. Oncology phase II trials generally use intermediate end-points such as tumor response or progression-free survival. The biomarker candidates can be evaluated in randomized phase II trials to maximize the new-treatment-versus-control-treatment difference, although this may require much larger sample size than is typical for phase II trials. In many phase II oncology clinical trials, tumor response is used as the end-point in a single-arm design and the candidate biomarkers evaluated to maximize the response rate. Although this approach may identify a subset of patients who respond better to both the new treatment and the control, it is a satisfactory approach if one is trying to find a subset of patients who have a nonnegligible response rate to the new treatment.

In some cases, the patient population is partitioned into distinct strata by the genomic classification and the purpose of the phase II trial is to determine in which strata the new drug has nonnegligible antitumor activity. This can be most easily accomplished by conducting a two-stage phase II design for the drug in each stratum (Simon, 1989, 470). The optimal two-stage design has been widely used in oncology for testing the null hypothesis that a new drug or regimen has a response probability of $\leq p_0$ versus the alternative that the response probability is $\geq p_1$, while maintaining a false positive error rate of $\leq \alpha$ and a false negative error rate of $\leq \beta$. Accrual terminates after the first stage if results are not consistent with a response rate $\geq p_1$. Otherwise, the second stage of accrual is completed.

Puszai, Anderson, and Hess (2007, 588) proposed a design illustrated in Figure 3.1 for evaluating a new drug based on objective tumor response when there are one or more binary candidate predictive biomarkers. The first stage of the trial is designed as the first stage of a traditional optimal two-stage design for evaluating the new drug overall for all patients regardless of marker status. Optimal two-stage designs can be computed using the Web-based program at http://brb.nci.nih.gov/. The first stage is defined by the number of patients (n_1) and the maximum number of responses (r_1) that would not warrant continuing the trial. After n_1 total patients are evaluable for response, if the number of responses is greater than r_1, then the drug is viewed as broadly promising enough to continue the phase II trial based on overall analysis not stratified by marker values. Accrual continues until a total of n_2 patients are evaluable. At that point, if the total number of responses is greater than r_2, then the drug is considered broadly active for that tumor type; otherwise, the drug is not considered broadly active. In either case, the trial is complete. If, however, the total number of responses in the initial n_1 patients is r_1 or less, then one initiates new phase II studies for each marker stratum of patients. One can count the patients already accrued as part of the initial stages of marker-stratified studies.

Jones and Holmgren (2007, 712) describe a phase II design for evaluating a new drug with a single candidate binary predictive biomarker. Specified numbers of marker-positive and marker-negative patients are

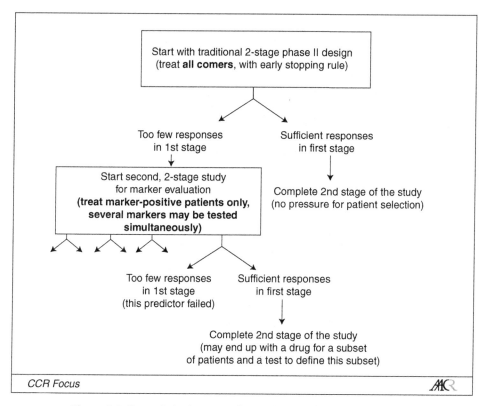

Figure 3.1. Pusztai, Anderson and Hess (2007) phase II design for evaluating the activity of a new drug and its relationship to the levels of one or more candidate binary biomarkers in a disease with binary response. If the drug is active overall in the initial stage of accrual, then separate evaluation in subsets determined by the biomarkers is not performed.

accrued in the first stage. If the first stage results suggest that the drug is active only in marker-positive patients, then the trial is completed with further accrual of marker-positive patients. If the first-stage results suggest that the drug is active for both marker-positive and marker-negative patients, then the trial is completed with further accrual of patients unrestricted by marker status. If the first-stage results suggest that the drug is inactive in both marker-positive and marker-negative patients, then the trial is terminated with no further accrual. The trial cutoff values and sample sizes are determined to preserve type I error and maximize power.

Freidlin et al. (2012) developed a design for a randomized phase II trial with time-to-event endpoint and a single binary biomarker. The design evaluates activity of the drug in both marker negative and marker positive strata.

In some cases, there is a single candidate predictive biomarker, and one expects that patients with larger values of the marker should be more responsive to the drug, but there is no inherent cut-point for positivity of that marker. Assume that there are K candidate cut -points $b_1, b_2, \ldots \ldots,$ b_K for the biomarker. The candidate cut points can be qualitative scores as in immunohistochemistry scoring, or they may be quantiles of a quantitative score (e.g., 25th percentile, median, and 75th percentile). Assume that the new drug is used as a single agent and objective response or degree of tumor shrinkage is used as the end-point. Let p_k denote the probability of response for patients with biomarker levels less than or equal to b_k and assume $p_1 \leq p_2 \leq \cdots \leq p_K$. One could conduct a phase II trial in a two-stage or multistage manner. For example, after accruing n_1 total patients, unrestricted with regard to biomarker level, one could test the hypothesis $H_{0i} : p_i \geq p^*$, where p^* is a response rate of interest. If there is no marker level i for which this hypothesis can be rejected at a prespecified significance level, then the trial continues accruing patients. Otherwise, second-stage accrual would be restricted to patients with markers above the largest level i^* for which the hypothesis was rejected. A Bayesian model could alternatively be used to restrict accrual.

A logistic regression model-based analysis can be used in the general case for relating the probability of an objective response to the values of multiple candidate biomarkers (e.g., degree of protein expression, presence or absence of gene amplification, and presence or absence of gene mutation). For example,

$$p(\underline{x}) = \frac{\exp\{\alpha + \underline{\beta}\underline{x}\}}{1 + \exp\{\alpha + \underline{\beta}\underline{x}\}} \tag{3.1}$$

where $\underline{x}$ denotes the vector of candidate biomarkers. For binary bio-markers, $x_i = 0$ or $x_i = 1$. For semiquantitative biomarkers with multiple levels, x_i denotes the level – again, with $x_i = 0$ denoting the lowest level. $\underline{\beta}$ denotes the vector of regression coefficients, with β_i representing the slope for the *i*th marker. More complicated models can be used to avoid the assumption of linearity for the effect of each quantitative or semiquantitative marker. $p(\underline{x})$ denotes the probability of response, for a patient with covariate vector $\underline{x}$, and α is the intercept of the model. Such a model enables one to evaluate the relationship of biomarker variables to response rate and to determine which candidate biomarker is most useful for predicting response. If there are multiple candidate markers but a single marker classifier is desired for use in the phase III trial, then in optimizing the fit of model (3.1) with regard to the regression coefficients, one would restrict attention to parameter vectors $\underline{\beta}$ for which only one component is nonzero.

The phase II trial should ideally be sized to enable such a model as (3.1) to be effectively used for selecting the best candidate and cut-point for use in the phase III trial. The required sample size will generally be driven by the number of responses to observe but will also depend on the number of candidate markers, the number of levels of each marker, and the correlation among the markers. Because of the complexity of the objective and the number of parameters involved, sample size planning may require simulation of the particular clinical trial being planned.

If time to progression is the end-point or if objective response is the end-point but the new drug is given in combination with standard chemotherapy, then a single-arm uncontrolled trial does not provide an estimate of the effect of the new drug. For example, one biomarker stratum might have a higher objective response rate to a combination than another stratum because the patients in one stratum respond better to the standard chemotherapy. Similarly, one biomarker stratum might have longer progression-free survival than another after single-agent treatment with the new drug because the biomarker influences outcome regardless of the treatment used. Consequently, in a phase II study of a new drug in combination with standard chemotherapy, it is desirable to use a control arm consisting of the standard chemotherapy alone. For such a trial, an appropriate model for analysis might be

$$p(\underline{x}) = \frac{\exp\{\alpha_0 + \alpha_1 z + \underline{\beta}\,\underline{x} + z\underline{\gamma}\,\underline{x}\}}{1 + \exp\{\alpha_0 + \alpha_1 z + \underline{\beta}\,\underline{x} + z\underline{\gamma}\,\underline{x}\}} \qquad (3.2)$$

instead of (3.1). $p(\underline{x})$ still denotes the probability of response for a patient with a vector of biomarkers $\underline{x}$. In (3.2), z denotes a binary treatment indicator (0 for the control group, 1 for the regimen containing the new drug). $\underline{\beta}$ is the vector of prognostic regression coefficients that reflect the effect of the candidate markers on response for both the new regimen and the control. $\underline{\gamma}$ is the vector of predictive regression coefficients that reflect the effect of the candidate markers on response for the new regimen over and above the prognostic effect.

When the end-point is progression-free survival in a randomized phase II clinical trial, then model (3.2) may be replaced by a proportional hazards model

$$\log \left(\frac{h(t, \underline{x}, z)}{h_0(t)} \right) = \alpha_1 z + \underline{\beta}\,\underline{x} + z\underline{\gamma}\,\underline{x} \qquad (3.3)$$

where $h(t, \underline{x}, z)$ denotes the hazard function at time t for a patient with treatment indicator z and vector of candidate markers $\underline{x}$. Proportional hazards models are popular because the regression coefficients can be determined without specifying the baseline hazard function $h_0(t)$.

Bayesian adaptive designs have been proposed for randomized phase II trials with multiple treatment arms and multiple candidate biomarkers. Randomized phase II trials involving multiple new regimens may be difficult to organize, however, because the drugs may come from different companies. Such trials can be efficient if there is a control arm that can be shared among the new treatment arms. A Bayesian adaptive design was used for the BATTLE I clinical trial in advanced non–small cell lung cancer (Kim & Simon, 2011, 830). Four treatment regimens were evaluated; no control group was used and the end-point was whether or not the patient had disease progression by eight weeks after start of treatment. The four treatments were erlotinib, vandetanib, sorafenib, and the combination of erlotinib plus bexarotene. Patients were stratified into four marker strata: (1) patients with mutations or overexpression of EGFR; (2) patients with KRAS or BRAF mutations; (3) patients with overexpression of VEGF; and (4) patients with overexpression of RXR or Cyclin D1. The last stratum contained only 6 of a total of 244 randomized patients. Ideally one would like to know enough about the drug being developed that one could define one or a small

Table 3.1. *BATTLE-1 Results*

Marker group	Erlotinib	Vandetanib	Erlotinib + bexarotene	Sorafenib	Total
EGFR	6/17 (35%)	11/27 (41%)	11/20 (55%)	9/23 (39%)	37/87 (43%)
KRAS–BRAF	1/7 (14%)	0/3 (0%)	1/3 (33%)	11/14 (79%)	13/27 (48%)
VEGF–VEGFR-2	10/25 (40%)	6/16 (38%)	0/3 (0%)	25/39 (64%)	41/83 (49%)
RXR–CyclinDl	0/1 (0%)	0/0 (NA)	1/1 (100%)	1/4 (25%)	2/6 (33%)
None	3/8 (38%)	0/6 (0%)	5/9 (56%)	11/18 (61%)	19/41 (46%)
Total	20/58 (34%)	17/52 (33%)	18/36 (50%)	57/98 (58%)	112/244 (46%)

Note: Eight-week disease control status by treatment and marker groups.
Source: Kim et al. 2011, *Cancer Discovery*, Table 2.

number of candidate predictive biomarkers related to the targets of the drug. In BATTLE I, the same biomarker candidates were used for all four treatment arms. Since Erlotinib is a small molecule inhibitor of EGFR, the use of EGFR mutation or overexpression as candidate markers makes sense, although they were combined into one category in BATTLE. The other pairings of drugs and markers are less compelling as a basis for conducting a phase II trial.

The idea of the Bayesian adaptive approach is to start with assigning a treatment to a patient based on randomization with equal probability for receiving each of the four treatments and to modify the randomization weights as accumulating data indicate that some treatments appear more effective for some of the four biomarker strata. This can be reassuring to patients, although Korn and Freidlin have shown that outcome-adaptive treatment assignment requires a larger sample size to maintain the same statistical power as equal randomization (Korn & Freidlin, 2011, 831). Korn and Freidlin indicate that in some cases the total sample size is so substantially increased with adaptive randomization that the expected number of patients receiving the inferior treatments is also increased.

The results of the BATTLE trial are shown in Table 3.1 as the number of patients without progression at eight weeks divided by the number of patients treated. Eighty-seven of the 244 randomized patients were in the EGFR stratum. There was relatively little variability in the number of patients assigned to the four treatment arms in the EGFR stratum probably because all of the treatment arms appeared active. The

Table 3.2. *Optimal Two-Stage Designs with Type I and Type II Error Rates of 20%*

P_0	P_1	n_1	r_1	n_{tot}	r_{tot}	PET
0.30	0.60	3	0	8	3	0.34
0.30	0.55	5	1	14	5	0.53
0.35	0.60	5	1	12	5	0.43
0.35	0.55	11	3	19	8	0.53

Note: PET = probability of early termination.

KRAS–BRAF stratum contained only 27 patients, most of whom (14) received sorafenib. The number of patients in that stratum receiving vandetanib or erlotinib plus bexarotene is almost too low for evaluation, but the adaptive randomization was effective for assigning the majority of patients in the stratum to a regimen with substantial apparent activity. The VEGF stratum contained 83 of the 244 randomized patients. A substantial number of patients were randomized to erlotinib (25) and vandetanib (16), which were active with proportion without progression ratios of about 40%. The number of patients treated with erlotinib plus bexarotane appears too small for adequate evaluation of the treatment. Almost twice as many patients were assigned to sorafinib (39) as to each of the erlotinib and vandetanib arms, and 64% of the patients receiving sorafinib were without progression at eight weeks. One of the targets of sorafinib is VEGFR-2, so the 64% nonprogression rate in that stratum is not entirely surprising.

Hence the adaptive randomization appeared successful. The analysis used was not comparative. Each treatment arm was evaluated on its own relative to a fixed standard of 30% nonprogression at eight weeks. A treatment was considered promising for phase III trial in a biomarker stratum if there was more than an 80% posterior probability that the nonprogression ratio of the treatment in that stratum was greater than 30%.

A very simple alternative to the design used in BATTLE I might have been to conduct separate optimal two-stage phase II trials for each of the drug-biomarker combinations. Table 3.2 shows the parameters of two-stage designs for distinguishing a nonprogression rate of P_0 from a nonprogression rate of P_1 with type I and type II error rates of 20%.

The second stage is conducted if the number of patients without eight-week progression in the first stage exceeds r_1. If the second stage is conducted the total sample size is n_{tot} and the drug is considered inadequately active in that stratum if no more than r_{tot} non-progressions are observed. The probability of early termination after the first stage if the null hypothesis is true is given by the last column. For any of these optimal two-stage designs conducted for each of the four treatments in each of the three biomarker strata that accrued patients, the maximum sample size required would have been no greater than 12 * 19 = 228 patients, even if none of the strata stopped early. This is about the same as the 244 randomized patients in BATTLE.

Additional discussions of design considerations for phase II trials containing biomarkers are given by Fox, Curt, and Balis (2002, 305), McShane, Hunsberger, and Adjei (2009, 832), Beckman, Clark, and Chen (2011, 833), Freidlin et al. (2012), and Lai et al. (2012, 834).

4

Enrichment Designs

Predictive classifiers provide information about whether a particular patient is likely (or unlikely) to benefit from a particular treatment. One classic example is the level of expression of the estrogen receptor protein in breast cancer cells as a predictor of response to antiestrogen treatments such as tamoxifen. A more recent example is the level of expression of the Her2 protein or the degree of amplification of the Her2 gene in breast cancer cells as a predictor of response to the anti-Her2 antibody trastuzumab. After anti-EGFR antibodies cetuximab and panitumumab were approved for the treatment of advanced colorectal cancer, it was demonstrated that the drugs were not effective for patients whose tumors contained KRAS mutations. Hence KRAS mutation status is a (negative) predictive marker for the use of these antibodies in colorectal cancer. Whether a biomarker or classifier is predictive depends on the context of use, the treatment, the alternative available treatment and the class of patients. Predictive classifiers have generally been based on single-protein or single-gene measurements related to the mechanism of action of the drug. Predictive classifiers and predictive scores can, however, be multigene or multiprotein summaries of the contributions of multiple measurements. For example, in addition to its established role as a prognostic factor for patients with node-negative breast cancer, the TAILORx clinical trial will test the role of Oncotype DX recurrence score as a predictive factor for benefit from chemotherapy in node-positive patients (Sparano & Paik, 2008, 620).

Many cancer drugs are being developed today with companion diagnostics to be used as predictive biomarkers. Sawyers (2008, 683) has stated that "one of the main barriers to further progress is identifying the biological indicators, or biomarkers, of cancer that predict who will benefit from a particular targeted therapy." This increases the complexity of drug development and requires that an effective predictive biomarker be identified and a test for it be analytically validated prior to the launch of the phase III pivotal clinical trials of the drug. The discovery and phase II refinement of predictive biomarkers can be complex. It may require larger phase II databases, new approaches to phase II trial design as described in Chapter 3, or designs based on neo-adjuvant treatment (Pusztai, 2004, 641; Pusztai, Anderson, & Hess, 2007, 588; Hess et al., 2006, 637).

The objective of a phase III pivotal clinical trial is to evaluate whether a new drug, given in a defined manner, has medical utility for a defined set of patients. Pivotal trials test prespecified hypotheses about treatment effectiveness in specified patient population groups. The role of a predictive classifier is usually to prospectively specify the population of patients in whom the new treatment will be evaluated. By prospectively specifying the patient population in the protocol, one assures that adequate numbers of such patients are available, and avoids the problems of post hoc subset analysis. The process of classifier development may be exploratory and subjective based on data collected prior to the phase III trial, but the use of the classifier in the phase III trial should not be.

Figure 4.1 shows a design in which a classifier is used to define eligibility for a randomized clinical trial comparing a new drug to a control regimen. This approach was used for the development of trastuzumab. Patients with metastatic breast cancer whose tumors expressed Her2 at a 2+ or 3+ level based on an immunohistochemistry test were eligible for randomization (Slamon et al., 2001, 596). The clinical trial randomized 469 patients, but the number whose tumors were tested was not stated. If approximately 75% of patients had available specimens and adequate tests and 25% of patients with adequate tests were Her2 positive, then about 2,500 patients would have been screened to obtain 469 eligible for randomization.

Simon and Maitournam (2005, 495; 2006, 494) and Maitournam and Simon (2005, 387) studied the efficiency of this approach relative to

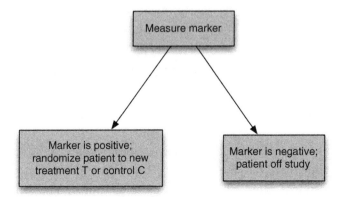

Figure 4.1. Enrichment design or targeted enrichment design. Patients are screened using a diagnostic test and prespecified cut-point for positivity. Test-positive patients are included in the randomized clinical trial comparing a new treatment to an appropriate control. Test-negative patients are excluded from the clinical trial.

the standard approach of randomizing all patients without measuring the marker. They determined the number of patients one must randomize for each design to have a specified statistical power for rejecting the null hypothesis at a specified statistical significance level. They assumed that there was a treatment effect of size δ_+ for the test-positive patients and a treatment effect δ_- for the test-negative patients. With the enrichment design, the biomarker test is used to screen the patients, and so the null hypothesis is tested only on the test-positive patients. They accrue n_E test-positive patients, where n_E is determined to have power $1 - \beta$ for rejecting the null hypothesis in the test-positive patients at statistical significance level α. The size of the treatment effect in the test-positive patients is δ_+. For the standard design, n_S unscreened patients are randomized to have power $1 - \beta$ for the test of the null hypothesis. In the unscreened patients, however, the size of the treatment effect is approximately

$$\text{prev}\,\delta_+ + (1 - \text{prev})\,\delta_-$$

where prev denotes the proportion of patients who are test positive. If δ_- is much less than δ_+, then this average treatment effect in the unscreened population will be much less than δ_+, and to have power $1 - \beta$ in both cases, one will have n_E much less than n_S.

For binary end-points, Simon and Maitournam found that the relative efficiency of the standard design relative to the enrichment design is approximately

$$n_S/n_E \approx \left[\delta_+ / (\text{prev}\delta_+ + (1 - \text{prev})\delta_-) \right]^2 . \qquad (4.1)$$

They computed the relative efficiency of the two designs using a more exact formula, but the preceding approximation was accurate when the response rates were not too close to 0 or 1. The same approximation is also relevant to the survival end-point setting, where n_E and n_S are interpreted as number of events rather than number of patients.

In cases in which the new treatment is completely ineffective in test-negative patients, $\delta_- = 0$, the preceding formula simplifies to

$$n_S/n_E \approx 1/\text{prev}^2 \text{ when } \delta_- = 0.$$

Hence, if half the patients are test positive and the new treatment is completely ineffective in test-negative patients, then the standard design requires four times as many randomized patients as the enrichment design.

Often, however, it is unrealistic to expect that the treatment will be completely ineffective for test-negative patients. The treatment may have some effectiveness for test-negative patients either because the assay is imperfect for measuring deregulation of the putative molecular target or because the drug has off-target effects. Because these alternatives cannot generally be distinguished, there is little value in decomposing δ_- into these components. If the new treatment is half as effective in test-negative patients as in test-positive patients, $\delta_- = \delta_+/2$, then the right-hand side of expression (4.1) simplifies to

$$n_S/n_E = 4/(\text{prev} + 1)^2 \text{ if } \delta_- = \delta_+/2.$$

If prev $= 0.5$, then n_S/n_E equals about 1.77 when 50% of the patients are test positive. Under these conditions, the standard design requires about 77% more patients than the enrichment design. If only 25% of the patients are test positive, then the ratio is 2.56, and the standard design requires two and a half times as many patients as the enrichment design. As the prevalence of test positivity decreases, the advantage of the enrichment design relative to the standard design increases because the treatment effect for the unselected population becomes more drastically diluted by the dominant number of test-negative patients for whom the treatment effect is smaller.

When fewer than half of the patients are test positive and the new treatment is relatively ineffective in test-negative patients, the number of randomized patients required for an enrichment design is often dramatically smaller than the number of randomized patients required for a standard design. This was the case for trastuzumab. The enrichment design that led to approval of trastuzumab was conducted in 469 patients with metastatic breast cancer whose tumors overexpressed Her2 based on immunohistochemical analysis in a central laboratory. The results were highly significant with regard to several end-points, including one-year survival rate (78% vs. 67%). The trial of 469 patients provides 90% power for detecting a 13.5% improvement in the one-year survival rate above a baseline of 67% with a two-sided 5% significance level. If benefit from the drug were limited to the 25% of patients expected to be test positive, then the overall improvement in one-year survival rate would be only 3.375% for a standard design, and a total of about 8,050 patients would be required for 90% power to detect such a small effect. This is 17.2 times as many patients as for the enrichment design, in good agreement with the ratio of 16 computed from the approximate form of equation (4.1). If the test-negative patients benefit half as much as the test-positive patients, then 1,254 total patients would be required for 90% power with the standard design. This is 2.7 times as many for the enrichment design, but is much less than the number required for screening with the enrichment design.

Simon and Maitournam also compared the enrichment design to the standard design with regard to the number of screened patients. For the standard design, the test is not used for screening, but to obtain

n_E test-positive patients for randomization in the enrichment design, one must screen approximately n_E/prev patients. If we use the notation $n'_E = n_E/\text{prev}$ to denote the number of screened patients for the enrichment design and plug this into (4.1), we obtain

$$n_S/n'_E \approx \text{prev} \left[\delta_+ / \left(\text{prev}\delta_+ + (1 - \text{prev})\delta_- \right) \right]^2 \qquad (4.2)$$

for the ratio of number of randomized patients for the standard design to number of screened patients for the enrichment design. When $\delta_- = 0$, this reduces to $1/\text{prev}$, which is always greater than 1, indicating that in this situation, the number of randomized patients for the standard design is always greater than the number of screened patients for the enrichment design. When $\delta_- = \delta_+/2$, equation (4.2) reduces to

$$n_S/n'_E = 4\text{prev}/(\text{prev} + 1)^2 \ \text{ if } \ \delta_- = \delta_+/2,$$

which is not always greater than 1. If prev $= 0.5$, then the ratio equals 8/9. In this case, the standard design requires about 77% more patients than the enrichment design randomizes, but the enrichment design has to screen about 12% more patients than the standard design randomizes. If prev $= 0.25$, then the ratio equals approximately 0.64. In this case, the standard design randomizes 2.56 more patients than the enrichment design, but the enrichment design screens about a third more patients than the standard design randomizes.

Some authors have mistakenly claimed that the derivations of Simon and Maitournam were based on the assumption that the test was perfect. This was not the case. As mentioned earlier, in these derivations, the treatment effect in test-negative patients incorporated both the inaccuracy of the test and the lack of specificity of the treatment. The treatment effect can be decomposed in the following way. Let Δ_+ and Δ_- denote the treatment effects in patients whose disease is biologically marker positive and marker negative, respectively. Let sens and spec denote the sensitivity and specificity of the test for identifying these two types of diseases, respectively, and let γ_+ denote the proportion of cases that are biologically marker positive. Let TE denote having a treatment effect.

Table 4.1. *Sample Data Relating Test Threshold to Sensitivity and Specificity for Identifying a Deregulated Pathway*

Threshold	Sensitivity	Specificity
Low	0.95	0.6
Middle	0.8	0.8
High	0.6	0.95

Then we can express δ_+, δ_-, and prev in terms of these parameters. For example,

$$
\begin{aligned}
\delta_+ &= \Pr[\text{TE}|\text{test+}] \\
&= \frac{\Pr[\text{TE, test+}]}{\Pr[\text{test+}]} \\
&= \frac{\Pr[\text{TE, test + }|\text{disease+}]\Pr[\text{disease+}] + \Pr[\text{TE, test + }|\text{disease} -]\Pr[\text{disease} -]}{\Pr[\text{test + }|\text{disease+}]\Pr[\text{disease+}] + \Pr[\text{test + }|\text{disease} -]\Pr[\text{disease} -]} \\
&= \frac{\Delta_+ \text{sens}\, \gamma_+ + \Delta_-(1 - \text{spec})(1 - \gamma_+)}{\text{sens}\, \gamma_+ + (1 - \text{spec})(1 - \gamma_+)}.
\end{aligned}
$$

Similarly,

$$
\delta_- = \frac{\Delta_- \text{spec}(1 - \gamma_+) + \Delta_+(1 - \text{sens})\gamma_+}{\text{spec}(1 - \gamma_+) + (1 - \text{sens})\gamma_+}
$$

$$
\text{prev} = \text{sens}\gamma_+ + (1 - \text{spec})(1 - \gamma_+).
$$

These relationships permit one to evaluate how test performance and treatment specificity separately influence the efficiency of the enrichment design. They can be used to optimize the threshold of positivity used for an enrichment design if data are available on how sensitivity and specificity depend on that threshold. Suppose, for example, that three thresholds were being considered and that the estimated sensitivities and specificities of the test were as shown in Table 4.1. If the treatment is completely ineffective for patients with biologically marker-negative disease ($\Delta_- = 0$), then the preceding relationships become

$$
\delta_+ = \Delta_+\gamma_+ \text{sens}/\text{prev}
$$

$$
\delta_- = \Delta_+\gamma_+(1 - \text{sens})/(1 - \text{prev}) \tag{4.3}
$$

where sensitivity and prevalence vary with the threshold. With the assumption that $\Delta_- = 0$, the treatment effects in test-positive and test-negative patients depend on the specificity of the test because the prevalence does. Expression (4.1) can be rewritten as

$$n_S/n_E \approx \left(\frac{\text{sens}}{\text{prev}}\right)^2. \tag{4.4}$$

If we assume that the proportion of patients with biologically marker-positive disease is 50%, then for the low threshold, the prevalence of test positivity will be 0.95 * 0.5 + 0.4 * 0.5 = 0.675. For the intermediate threshold, the prevalence of test positivity will be 0.8 * 0.5 + 0.2 * 0.5 = 0.5, and for the high threshold, the prevalence will be 0.6 * 0.5 + 0.05 * 0.5 = 0.375. Using expression (4.4), the randomization ratio for the low threshold is 1.98. So for the low threshold, about 67.5% of the patients will be test positive, and the standard design will require about twice as many patients as the enrichment design. For the intermediate threshold, half of the patients will be test positive, and the randomization ratio is 2.56, so it is somewhat more efficient than the low threshold in terms of number of patients required to randomize. For the high threshold, only 37.5% of the patients will be test positive, and the randomization ratio is again 2.56.

The intermediate threshold will require fewer screened patients than the high threshold and therefore seems optimal.

Focusing initial development on test-positive patients can lead to clarity in determining who benefits from the drug. If the enrichment design establishes that the drug is effective in test-positive patients, the drug could be later developed in test-negative patients. This is preferable to testing new drugs in uncharacterized heterogeneous populations, resulting in false-negative results for the overall population.

The methods of sample size planning for the design of enrichment trials are available online at http://brb.nci.nih.gov/. The Web-based programs are available for binary and survival–disease-free survival endpoints. The planning takes into account the performance characteristics of the tests and specificity of the treatment effects. The programs provide comparisons to standard nonenrichment designs based on the number of randomized patients required and the number of patients needed for screening to obtain the required number of randomized patients.

Further discussion and evaluation of the enrichment design is provided by Hoering et al. (2008), Sargent et al. (2005), Simon (2008b) and Mandrekar and Sargent (2009, 2010).

5

Including Both Test-Positive and Test-Negative Patients

When a predictive classifier has been developed but there is not compelling biological or phase II data that test negative patients do not benefit from the new treatment, it is generally best to include both classifier positive and classifier negative patients in the phase III clinical trials comparing the new treatment to the control regimen. In this case, it is essential that (i) an analysis plan be predefined in the protocol for how the predictive classifier will be used in the analysis, and (ii) the clinical trial be sized for adequate power for analysis of test-positive patients separately. It is not sufficient to just stratify, that is, balance, the randomization with regard to the classifier without specifying a complete analysis plan and sizing the trial appropriately. In fact, the main importance of stratifying the randomization is that it assures that only patients with adequate test results will enter the trial.

For phase III trials of a new treatment and prespecified binary classifier, the purpose of the trial is to evaluate the new treatment and to determine how treatment effectiveness depends on the prespecified classifier. The purpose is not to modify or optimize the classifier. If the classifier is a composite gene expression–based classifier, the purpose of the study is not to reexamine the contributions of each gene. If one does any of this, then an additional phase III trial may be needed to evaluate treatment benefit in subsets determined by the new classifier. In the following sections, I describe several analysis strategies for clinical trials that include patients positive and negative for a prespecified binary classifier. Such strategies are discussed in greater detail by Simon (2008a, 623; 2008b, 640).

The paradigm I employ for analysis of clinical trials involving one or more candidate biomarkers involves two components. The first is a test of the global null hypothesis that the treatment is uniformly ineffective. Testing the global null hypothesis at the 5% significance level ensures that the study-wise type I error rate is no greater than 5%. For studies involving prospective use of genomics, the test statistic for this null hypothesis may not be the conventional statistic of the difference in average effect between the treatment and control group; rather, it may be selected for sensitivity to the types of biomarker-specific treatment effects that are expected. The paradigm I shall use has a second component. If the study-wise null hypothesis is rejected, then we need to develop an *indication classifier* that identifies the biomarker-based characteristics of the patients for whom the new treatment should be used. Development of this indication classifier may or may not involve statistical significance testing. A statistical significance test of the global null hypothesis is the appropriate technology for preserving the studywise type I error. Development of an indication classifier is not necessarily a significant testing problem, particularly in complex settings with multiple candidate classifiers or unknown thresholds of positivity.

In this chapter, I consider the simple situation where there is a single candidate classifier and where a threshold distinguishing positivity from negativity has been prospectively specified. In cases in which one does not expect the treatment to be effective in the test-negative patients unless it is effective in the test-positive patients, the statistic used for testing the study-wise null hypothesis test might just be the p value for treatment effect within the test-positive patients. Letting p^* denote the test statistic for the study-wise test,

$$p^* = p_+. \tag{5.1}$$

If the treatment difference in test-positive patients is significant at the 5% level, then an indication classifier might be defined simply in the following way. The test-positive patients would be *indication classifier positive* and the test-negative patients would be considered indication positive if the treatment effect within the test-negative patients were statistically significant at the 0.05 level. The 0.05 level can be used because the type I error of the trial has already been protected by the initial test.

If p^* is not significant at the 0.05 level, then the treatment is considered ineffective for all patients. Liu et al. (2010, 679) modify this approach to delay accrual of any test-negative patients until interim results in test-positive patients suggest that the new treatment is promising for that stratum.

The analysis plan described in the previous paragraph is for situations in which one has great confidence that the test-negative patients will not benefit from the treatment unless the test-positive patients do. At the other extreme is the situation in which one has very limited a priori confidence in the predictive marker and uses it for a fallback analysis. Simon and Wang (2006, 499) proposed an analysis plan in which the new treatment group is first compared to the control group overall. If that difference is not significant at a reduced significance level such as 0.03, then the new treatment is compared to the control group just for test-positive patients. The latter comparison uses a threshold of significance of 0.02 or whatever portion of the traditional 0.05 is not used by the initial test. For the paradigm used here, the single study-wise null hypothesis can have a rejection region based on

$$p_{ave} < \alpha_{ave} \text{ or } p_+ < \alpha_+ \tag{5.2}$$

where p_{ave} represents the p value for average treatment effect for all randomized patients and p_+ denotes the p value for treatment effect in the test-positive patients. Variable p_{ave} might be based on a traditional null hypothesis test of all randomized patients, ignoring the biomarker, or it might be a test that includes all patients but is stratified by biomarker value. The critical values α_{ave} and α_+ must be selected so that the type I error is preserved at 5% when the uniform null hypothesis is true. If the study-wise null hypothesis is rejected, an indication classifier should be developed.

In this simple situation with a single binary classifier, it seems strange to talk about development of an indication classifier. Usually we think of making inferences about treatment effects in subsets and utilize multiple inference procedures for structuring and evaluating the inferences. In more complex settings with markers without predefined thresholds and with multiple candidate markers, the multiple inference framework is inadequate. It results in using indication for treatment policies that either treat everyone or no one – policies that do not have good performance characteristics in terms of their overtreatment or undertreatment of future patients. Here we recommend using the indication classifier paradigm and directly evaluating the performance characteristics of an indication classifier for benefiting future patients. These performance characteristics can be evaluated using resampling methods as described later. For the current situation, the classifier impicit in the usual clinical trial without prespecified biomarker might be to use the treatment for all patients if $p_{ave} < 0.05$, and if not, then to use the new treatment for no patients. The fallback analysis plan proposed by Simon and Wang recommends the treatment for all patients if p_{ave} is less than some reduced level α_{ave}. If $p_{ave} > \alpha_{ave}$ and $p_+ < 0.05 - \alpha_{ave}$ then the new treatment is recommended for test-positive patients. If neither of these conditions is true, then the new treatment is not recommended at all. Wang, O'Neill, and Hung (2007, 584), Song and Chi (2007, 583), and Zhao, Dmitrienko, and Tamura (2010, 839) have utilized the correlation between the overall test and the subset test to refine the threshold p values used for the two tests to give greater statistical power. Simon (2008b) discusses the analysis strategies described here.

5.1 Interaction Tests

The traditional approach to the "two-way analysis of variance" problem is to first test whether there is a significant interaction between the effect of one factor (treatment) and the second factor (biomarker). If the interaction test is not significant, then the treatment effect is evaluated overall, not within levels of the second factor. If the interaction test is significant, then treatment effect is evaluated separately within the levels of the second factor (e.g., test-positive and test-negative classes). This is similar to the approach proposed by Sargent et al. (2005, 450). In fact, Sargent et al. called the design containing both test-positive and test-negative patients an interaction design. This corresponds to using a study-wise test statistic

$$p^* = (\text{Ind} \, (p_{int} \leq \alpha_{int})) \, p_+ + (1 - \text{Ind} \, (p_{int} \leq \alpha_{int})) \, p_{ave}. \quad (5.3)$$

The indicator function Ind ($p_{\text{int}} \leq \alpha_{\text{int}}$) equals 1 if the p value for interaction is less than or equal to a threshold α_{int}. If that is the case, then the hypothesis test for the study is based on the p value for treatment effect in the test-positive patients; otherwise, the indicator function is zero and the hypothesis test for the study is based on the p value for the average treatment effect for all patients.

If $p^* < 0.05$, then one needs to develop an indication classifier. A natural classifier might be to recommend the treatment for all patients if the interaction test is not significant at level α_{int} and $p_{\text{ave}} < 0.05$. If the interaction test is significant at level α_{int} and $p_+ < 0.05$, but $p_- > 0.05$, then the treatment is recommended only for the test-positive patients.

Testing for interaction is not the purpose of the clinical trial. The purpose of the trial is to compare the new treatment to the control in test-positive and test-negative subsets. The interaction test serves only to define the test statistic for the test of the study-wise null hypothesis and perhaps for structuring an indication classifier. Since the interaction test will often have inadequate statistical power, it may not serve well as a basis for defining an indication classifier that will serve future patients well. It can require substantially more patients to test for interaction at the two-sided 5% significance level than for the analysis plans described here. For our purpose, the interaction test should be one-sided and performed at a threshold above the traditional 5% level. The significance level threshold at which the interaction test is performed should reflect the degree evidence available at the start of the trial that treatment benefit, if it exists at all, will be limited to test-positive patients. The traditional two-sided 5% significance threshold is only appropriate for traditional post hoc data subset analysis settings in which there is very limited a priori evidence for a major difference in treatment effect among subsets. When the a priori evidence is very strong, one might think of the threshold as being 1.0; that is, the treatment effect is automatically evaluated separately for the test-positive and test-negative subsets.

5.2 Probabilistic Indication Classifier

Karuri and Simon (2012, 826) developed a Bayesian design for a randomized clinical trial with a single binary classifier. They develop a two-stage randomized design for comparing a new treatment to control. At the end of the first stage, they perform an interim futility analysis for determining whether accrual should be stopped for test-negative patients or for all patients or whether accrual should be continued in both strata. They introduce a class of joint prior distributions for the treatment effect in test-negative and test-positive patients that enables one to reflect the degree of prior evidence that exists for the hypothesis that the new treatment is unlikely to benefit test-negative patients, particularly if it does not benefit test-positive patients. The interim futility analysis utilizes this joint prior and hence may serve to better protect test-negative patients from continuing to be exposed to an investigational treatment that is not expected to benefit them.

The results of Karuri and Simon can be used for developing an indication classifier even if their two-stage Bayesian design is not used. We let δ_+ and δ_- denote the true treatment effect in test-positive and test-negative patients, respectively. One must specify a joint prior distribution for δ_+ and δ_- that reflects the degree of prior confidence one has in the classifier for identifying the patients who are likely to benefit from the new treatment. Karuri and Simon described a family of prior distributions parameterized by three parameters p_{00}, r_1, and r_2:

$$\Pr[\delta_+ = \delta_- = 0] = p_{00}$$
$$\Pr[\delta_- = 0 | \delta_+ = \delta^*] = r_1 \qquad (5.4)$$
$$\Pr[\delta_+ = 0 | \delta_- = \delta^*] = r_2.$$

Karuri and Simon utilized a four-point joint prior in which, for each test subset, the treatment effect is either 0 or δ^*, the latter representing treatment effect of clinical importance. A model with strong a priori confidence in the classifier is represented by a small value of r_2; you expect the treatment to work for test-positive patients if it works for test-negative patients; that is, the treatment is likely only to work for test-negative patients if it works in test-positive patients. Strong confidence in the classifier may also mean that you do not expect the treatment to work in test-negative patients even if it works in test-positive patients, so r_1 would be large. With very limited confidence in the classifier, r_1

and r_2 would be small because you would expect the treatment to work the same in both test-positive and test-negative cases.

At the end of the trial, based on the prior distribution specified at the start and on the observed treatment effect in each subset, one can compute the joint posterior distribution of δ_+ and δ_-. Suppose, for example, the observed treatment effects $(\hat{\delta}_+, \hat{\delta}_-)$ are independently normal with means δ_+ and δ_- with standard deviations s_+ and s_-. The probabilistic indication classifier is based on

$$\Pr[\delta_+ = \delta_- = 0 | \hat{\delta}_+, \hat{\delta}_-]$$
$$= c\phi(\hat{\delta}_+; 0, s_+)\phi(\hat{\delta}_-; 0, s_-) p_{00}$$
$$\Pr[\delta_+ = \delta^*, \delta_- = 0 | \hat{\delta}_+, \hat{\delta}_-] = c\phi(\hat{\delta}_+; \delta^*, s_+)\phi(\hat{\delta}_-; 0, s_-) p_{10} \qquad (5.5)$$
$$\Pr[\delta_+ = \delta^*, \delta_- = \delta^* | \hat{\delta}_+, \hat{\delta}_-] = c\phi(\hat{\delta}_+; \delta^*, s_+)\phi(\hat{\delta}_-; \delta^*, s_-) p_{11}$$
$$\Pr[\delta_+ = 0, \delta_- = \delta^* | \hat{\delta}_+, \hat{\delta}_-] = c\phi(\hat{\delta}_+; 0, s_1)\phi(\hat{\delta}_-; \delta^*, s_+) p_{01}$$

The normalization constant c is determined by the fact that these four probabilities must sum to 1. The factors such as $\phi(\hat{\delta}_+; 0, s_+)$ denote the normal density function for value $\hat{\delta}_+$ with mean 0 and standard deviation s_+. The factors such as $p_{10} = \Pr[\delta_+ = \delta^*, \delta_- = 0]$ are prior probabilities based on the assumed values of p_{00}, r_1, and r_2. After some algebra, one can show

$$p_{10} = \Pr[\delta_+ = \delta^*, \delta_- = 0] = r_1 \Pr[\delta_+ = \delta^*]$$
$$p_{01} = \Pr[\delta_+ = 0, \delta_- = \delta^*] = r_2 \Pr[\delta_- = \delta^*] \qquad (5.6)$$

The prior probability $p_{11} = \Pr[\delta_+ = \delta_- = \delta^*]$ can be computed by subtraction since the four prior probabilities must sum to 1. At the end of the trial, one can compute the four posterior probabilities shown in (5.5). One can then compute from these the marginal posterior probability that $\delta_+ = \delta^*$ and the marginal posterior probability that $\delta_- = \delta^*$.

These provide the posterior probabilities that the new treatment is more effective than control in the test-positive and test-negative patients, respectively. These two values provide useful information for a labeling indication of a drug and a tool for informing the treatment decisions of external physicians.

Indication classifiers are best evaluated interms of expected net outcome for a population of future patients if the classifier is used for
treatment selection. One should require that the analysis provide an
unbiased estimate of the true treatment effect in the indicator positive
population. We shall discuss in Chapter 8 how to use cross-validation
to obtain such an estimate. Cross-validation can also provide a proper
estimate of the expected treatment effect for the full population resulting
from the use of the indication classifier in the future.

5.3 Planning Sample Size

The most straightforward approach to planning sample size for the
clinical trial is to plan for having adequate statistical power for rejecting
the study-wise null hypothesis. For example, consider the case in which
the study-wise null hypothesis is tested using the test statistic $p^* = p_+$, as in
(5.1). The sample size must then be planned to have an adequate number
of patients or events for test-positive patients. To have 90% power in
the test-positive patients for detecting a 50% reduction in hazard for
the new treatment versus control at a one-sided 5% significance level
requires about 72 events among test-positive patients (see formula A.2
in Appendix A). In general, when n_+ test-positive patients are accrued,
there will be approximately n_+/prev total patients and approximately
$n_- = (1 - \text{prev})\, n_+/\text{prev}$ test-negative patients, where prev denotes the
proportion of test-positive patients. With a time-to-event end-point, at
the time that there are E_+ events in test-positive patients, there will be
approximately

$$E_- = E_+ \left(\frac{\lambda_-}{\lambda_+} \right) \left(\frac{1 - \text{prev}}{\text{prev}} \right) \tag{5.7}$$

events in the test-negative group. In expression (5.7), the symbols λ_- and
λ_+ denote the event rates in the test-negative and test-positive control
groups at the time that there are E_+ events in the test-positive group. As
earlier, prev represents the proportion of test-positive patients. If, at the
time of analysis, the event rates in the two strata are about equal, then
the ratio of lamdas will be about 1. If E_+ is 72 and if the prevalence of

test-positive patients is 0.25, then E_- will be approximately 216 at the time of analysis.

If one is using the study-wise test as in (5.2), the type I error can be controlled at 5% if $\alpha_{ave} + \alpha_+ = 0.05$. Wang, O'Neill, and Hung (2007, 584) have shown that the power of this approach can be improved by taking into account the correlation between p_{ave} and p_+. Song and Chi (2007, 583) also developed an approach that takes into account the correlation between the tests, but their method penalizes subset differences that are not accompanied by overall differences. This does not really seem appropriate for the prospective development of predictive biomarkers for molecularly targeted therapeutics. Whereas the conventional wisdom for interpreting clinical trial results was to ignore post hoc subset claims unless the overall effect was significant, this is inappropriate for focused prospective analysis of biomarkers and molecularly targeted agents.

To compute the power for testing the study-wise null hypothesis when (5.2) is employed, we will assume that a stratified analysis is used for computing p_{ave} based on $\hat{\delta}_{ave} = (E_+\hat{\delta}_+ + E_-\hat{\delta}_-)/(E_+ + E_-)$, where E_+ and E_- are the number of events in test-positive and test-negative patients, respectively. Under the uniform null hypothesis, $\hat{\delta}_{ave}$ is taken as approximately normal with mean zero and variance $4/(E_+ + E_-)$. To compute the power of the study-wise test of the global null hypothesis, we sampled values of $\hat{\delta}_+$ and $\hat{\delta}_-$ from independent normal distributions and computed $\hat{\delta}_{ave}$ and p_{ave}, as described. If one uses $\alpha_{ave} = 0.01$ and $\alpha_+ = 0.04$, then with 72 events in test-positive patients and 216 events in test-negative patients, there is approximately 89% power when there is a 50% reduction in hazard in the test-positive patients and no effect in the negatives. This slight drop in power compared to the use of the study-wise test (5.1) results from the use of $\alpha_+ = 0.04$ instead of 0.05. When there is a 33% reduction in hazard for both test-positive and test-negative patients, the power of the study-wide test is approximately 0.88. In these power calculations, we have assumed that the null hypothesis is rejected only if the new treatment does better than control; that is, p_{ave} and p_+ are computed with one-sided rejection regions.

When using test statistic (5.3) for evaluating the null hypothesis, some reduction in the values of α_{ave} and α_+ must be made to preserve the study-wise type I error. If one uses $\alpha_{int} = 0.10$, $\alpha_{ave} = 0.02$, and $\alpha_+ = 0.04$, then the type I error is 0.05. With 72 events in test-positive patients and 216 events in test-negative patients, the power is approximately 88%, when there is a 50% reduction in hazard in the test-positive patients and no effect in the negatives, and the power is approximately 92% when there is a uniform 33% reduction in hazard for both test-positive and test-negative patients.

Our perspective here has been that the purpose of the clinical trial is to test the global null hypothesis and to develop an indication classifier of the patients who benefit from the new treatment. Testing the null hypothesis that there is no interaction between treatment effect and test result does not have a direct role in this process unless the interaction test is part of the classifier definition. Interaction tests had a useful role in the era of exploratory subset analysis to protect against false claims of treatment effects when data dredging. For regulatory agencies that have to determine whether a test is necessary, the interaction test may be of relevance even with prospective trials focused on a single binary marker; therefore, we will explore here the sample size requirements for having adequate power for an interaction test.

With a time-to-event end-point (e.g., survival), testing the null hypothesis that $\delta_+ = \delta_-$ with power $1 - \beta$ for rejecting the null hypothesis when $\delta_+ = \delta^*$ and $\delta_- = 0$ at significance level α requires that the number of events in the test-positive and test-negative patients be chosen so that

$$\frac{1}{E_+^{int}} + \frac{1}{E_-^{int}} = \frac{1}{4}\left\{\frac{\delta^*}{k_{1-\alpha} + k_{1-\beta}}\right\}^2 \tag{5.8}$$

where the k values denote percentiles of the standard normal distribution. Alternatively, if we plan sample size to reject the uniform null hypothesis using test statistic (5.1) and require the same power $1 - \beta$ for rejecting the null hypothesis when $\delta_+ = \delta^*$ at the same significance level α, then the number of events required for test-positive patients is determined by

$$\frac{1}{E_+} = \frac{1}{4}\left\{\frac{\delta^*}{k_{1-\alpha} + k_{1-\beta}}\right\}^2. \tag{5.9}$$

If accrual is unrestricted by the test and if the event rates in test-positive and test-negative patients are the same at the time of the analysis, then $E_+ = \text{prev}\, E_{\text{tot}}$ and $E_+^{\text{int}} = \text{prev}\, E_{\text{tot}}^{\text{int}}$. Using these results with (5.8) and (5.9) gives

$$E_{\text{tot}}^{\text{int}} = E_{\text{tot}}/(1 - \text{prev}). \qquad (5.10)$$

For example, if 25% of patients are test positive, then prev = 0.25, and the number of total events needed to test the null hypothesis of no interaction is four-thirds times the number needed to test the null hypothesis of no treatment effect, that is, one-third more events. If the prevalence of test positivity is 50%, then twice as many events are needed to test the null hypothesis of no interaction. Web based programs for planning sample size for many of the designs described in this chapter are available at http://brb.nci.nih.gov.

5.4 Adaptively Modifying Types of Patients Accrued

Wang, O'Neill, and Hung (2007, 584) proposed a two-stage phase III design comparing a new treatment to a control, which starts with accruing both test-positive and test-negative patients. An interim analysis is performed evaluating the new treatment in the test-negative patients. If the observed efficacy for the control group exceeds that for the new treatment group and the difference exceeds a futility boundary, then accrual of test-negative patients terminates and accrual of additional test-positive patients is substituted for the unaccrued test-negative patients until the originally planned total sample size is reached. Wang, O'Neill, and Hung show computer simulations that indicate this design has greater statistical power than nonadaptive approaches.

The concept of curtailing accrual of test-negative patients based on an interim futility analysis can be implemented without the extension of trial duration resulting from substitution of test-positive for test-negative patients to achieve a prespecified total sample size. For example, the tests could be powered to detect a 50% reduction in hazard in test-positive patients and a 33% reduction in test-negative patients. If an interim analysis indicates futility for the test-negative patients, then accrual of test-negative patients may cease without affecting the target sample size or analysis for the test-positive patients.

A limitation of these approaches, however, is the conservativeness of futility boundaries. For example, Wang, O'Neill, and Hung (2007, 584) require that the futility boundary be in the region in which the observed efficacy is greater for the control group than for the new treatment group. Consequently, even if the new treatment is completely ineffective in the test-negative subset, the futility analysis will be successful less than half the time. The Bayesian two-stage design of Karuri and Simon (2012, 826) reduces this conservativeness by permitting the investigators to specify a prior distribution that reflects confidence in the test for identifying patients who are and are not likely to benefit from the new regimen. An interim analysis is performed after a prespecified number of events is observed and the posterior probabilities of treatment effect within test-negative and test-positive patients are computed based on the prior distribution specified at the outset and on events observed up until that point. If $\Pr[\hat{\delta}_+ = \delta^* | \text{interim data}]$ is not sufficiently large, then all accrual stops, and no claim of effectiveness is made. If that probability of effectiveness for test-positive patients is sufficiently large but $\Pr[\hat{\delta}_- = \delta^* | \text{interim data}]$ is too small, then accrual of negative patients stops but accrual of test-positive patients continues until the originally planned number of events in the test-positive patients is reached.

Liu et al. (2009, 679) proposed accruing only marker-positive patients during the initial stage. At the end of the first stage, an interim analysis is performed comparing outcome for the new treatment versus control for the marker-positive patients. If the results are not promising for the new treatment, then accrual stops and no treatment benefit is claimed. If the results are promising for the marker-positive patients at the end of the first stage, then accrual continues for marker-positive patients and also commences for marker-negative patients in the second stage.

These approaches use the same end-point for interim analysis as for final analysis. This will be adequate if the time to observing a patient's end-point is rapid relative to the accrual rate. For many oncology phase III trials using survival or disease-free survival, however, most of the patients would be accrued before a meaningful futility analysis based on sufficient events could be conducted, and these approaches would have to be modified to use an intermediate end-point for the interim futility analysis (Hunsberger, Zhao, & Simon, 2009, 840; Korn et al., 2012, 841).

6

Adaptive Threshold Design

Jiang, Freidlin, and Simon (2007, 345) described a "biomarker adaptive threshold design" for situations in which a predictive score or index is available at the start of the phase III trial, but a cut point for converting the score to a binary classifier is not established. With their design, tumor specimens are collected from all patients at entry, but the value of the predictive score is not used as an eligibility criterion. Their analysis plan does not stipulate that the assay for measuring the score needs to be performed prior to randomization, only prior to analysis.

We will present here a modification and extension of the design originally described by Jiang et al. Assume that there are K candidate thresholds or cut points $b_1, b_2, \ldots, b_K$ for the biomarker. Let l_K denote the log likelihood of the data computed assuming that there is a treatment effect restricted to patients with biomarker values greater than or equal to b_k. The test statistic for testing the null hypothesis of no treatment effect is

$$\max\{l_1, l_2, \ldots, l_K\}. \tag{6.1}$$

The null distribution of (6.1) is approximated by permuting the treatment labels, recalculating the $l_1, \ldots, l_K$ values and their maximum. This process is repeated for a thousand or more permutations of the treatment labels to approximate the distribution of the test statistic (6.1) under the null hypothesis that there is no relation of treatment with outcome regardless of marker level. From this permutation-based null distribution, one can determine the 95th percentile. That is the critical value for the test of the global null hypothesis that the new treatment is no better than control for any biomarker determined subset. If the value of (6.1) for the actual treatment labels is beyond that critical value for the null permutation distribution, then the global null hypothesis is rejected.

The null hypothesis tested above is not the usual null hypothesis of no average effect for all randomized patients. It is a *global null hypothesis* of no treatment effect for any of the biomarker-defined subsets. It is not a multiple testing approach, however; only one significance test is performed. It is a test that uses a test statistic that is sensitive to biomarker subset–specific treatment effects. Because multiple tests are not performed, there should be no concern about not having specified a cut point in advance. Often cut points are specified in advance based on inadequate data. Regulators sometimes prefer predefined cut points to ensure that the type I error rate is not inflated by multiple testing. On the other hand, the phase III trial generally provides more adequate data for establishing a cut point than do smaller phase II data sets, so long as the type I error rate is properly protected. The approach described here controls the type I error at 5% without specifying the cut point in advance.

If the global null hypothesis is rejected at the 5% significance level, then the next step is to develop an indication classifier that identifies the range of biomarker values that renders a patient a good candidate for the new treatment. Jiang, Freidlin, and Simon (2007, 345) develop a probabilistic indication classifier, which describes the probability that the patient would benefit from the new treatment as a function of the biomarker value. Probabilistic classifiers are useful for medical decision making because they provide information about which patients should clearly benefit from the new treatment, which would clearly not benefit, and for which there is more uncertainty. Although this may make medical decision making more complex, it enables physicians and patients to better tailor their decisions to their particular situations and preferences.

To obtain a probabilistic indication classifier, one might use a logistic model if the end-point is binary response or a proportional hazards model if the end-point is survival or disease-free survival. With a binary end-point, if the probability of response is determined by an unknown cut point, the logistic model relates the probability of response to biomarker level and treatment using

$$\log \left(\left(p(x, z) / (1 - p(z, x)) \right) = \alpha z + \beta x + \gamma I \left\{ x \geq b^* \right\} \right. \quad (6.2)$$

where p denotes the probability of response, z is a binary indicator of treatment ($z = 1$ for new treatment, $z = 0$ for control), x is the value of the single biomarker score, b^* is the unknown cut point for the biomarker score x, and I is the indicator function, which equals 1 when its argument is true and 0 otherwise. For a time-to-event end-point, the analogous proportional hazards model is

$$\log \left(h(z, x, k, t) / h_0(t) \right) = \alpha z + \beta x + \gamma I \left\{ x \geq b^* \right\} \qquad (6.3)$$

where h denotes the hazard of failure at time t. Model (6.2) or model (6.3) is maximized with regard to the parameters α, β, γ, b^* for the full data set. In performing the optimization, the optimal cut point b^* is only allowed to take values on the set of candidate cut points. Jiang et al. then take bootstrap samples of the observations and refit model (6.2) or (6.3) to obtain a bootstrap-based 95% confidence interval for the unknown cut point b^*. A bootstrap sample is obtained by sampling the cases with replacement, keeping the sample size the same as for the original data set. Let b_i^* denote the candidate cut point that maximizes log likelihood for the ith bootstrap sample. This is repeated for N bootstrap samples to obtain values $S = \left\{ b_1^*, \ldots, b_N^* \right\}$. For an individual with biomarker value x, let $F_S(x)$ denote the proportion of the elements in set S that are less than or equal to x. $F_S(x)$ is thus the "quantile" of x in the set S. $F_S(x)$ can be interpreted as the probability that $b^* \geq x$, that is, the probability that a patient with biomarker value x benefits from the new treatment. Consequently, $F_S(x)$ can be used as a probabilistic indication classifier.

The method of Karuri and Simon (2012, 826) can also be extended to provide a Bayesian probabilistic indication classifier. As in Karuri and Simon, we shall use a two-point prior for the treatment effect at any specified biomarker level b_k. Let $\delta(x)$ denote the treatment effect when the biomarker value is x. We assume that $\delta(x) = 0$ if x is less than the true cut point b^* and $\delta(x) = \delta^*$ otherwise. We also assume that a prior distribution for the threshold b^* is specified in advance. This prior generally will not be uniform on the candidate values $b_1, \ldots, b_K$. For example, the prior weight on b_1 indicates belief that the treatment is uniformly effective and the prior weight on b_K indicates belief that the treatment is uniformly ineffective.

Having specified the prior distribution in this way, at the end of the trial, one can compute the likelihood of the observed treatment effects at each marker level $\{\hat{\delta}(b_k), k = 1, \ldots, K\}$ and obtain the posterior distributions of the threshold b^*. More specifically, the joint posterior distribution can be approximated by

$$\Pr[b^* = b_k | \text{data}] = c\phi\left(\hat{\delta}_{<b_k}; 0, \sigma^2_{<b}\right)\phi\left(\hat{\delta}_{\geq b_k}; \delta^*, \sigma^2_{\geq b_k}\right) \qquad (6.4)$$
$$* \Pr[b^* = b_k]$$

where $\hat{\delta}_{<b_k}$ denotes the maximum likelihood estimate of the treatment effect for patients with biomarker $< b_k$, $\hat{\delta}_{\geq b_k}$ denotes the maximum likelihood estimate of the treatment effect for patients with biomarker $\geq b_k$, the $\sigma^2_{<b_k}$ and $\sigma^2_{\geq b_k}$ terms are the corresponding variances of these maximum likelihood estimates, ϕ denotes the normal density function, and c is a normalization constant that makes all the posterior probabilities sum to 1. The variances in this expression are obtained from the likelihood maximization but for survival data are approximately $4/E_{<b_k}$ and $4/E_{\geq b_k}$ based on the number of events less than and greater than or equal to the value of b_k respectively.

The Bayesian posterior distribution of b^* computed at the end of the clinical trial remains valid regardless of changes in patient eligibility based on interim findings. It can be used as a probabilistic indication classifier for labeling the recommended use of the new drug and for informing clinical decision making for future patients.

6.1 Sample Size Planning

In the previous chapter, we discussed planning a clinical trial with a pre-specified cut point having 72 test-positive patients and 216 test-negative patients (25% test positive) to provide 90% power for testing the null hypothesis using test statistic (6.1) of that chapter. Consequently, we simulated the trial design described here with exponentially distributed survival times, four candidate cut points, and a true treatment effect corresponding to a 50% reduction in hazard for the patients in the highest 25th percentile of the biomarker distribution and no treatment effect for the other patients. Rather than using the permutation test described earlier, we first simulated trials under the null hypothesis to obtain the upper 95th percentile of the maximized log likelihood ratio test statistic (6.1). In computing the maximized likelihood ratios, we required that the event rate for the new treatment be less than the control at the maximum, corresponding to a one-sided 5% significance level. We then simulated the trials under the alternative hypothesis that there was a 50% reduction in hazard for the top biomarker stratum (i.e., top 25th percentile with three interior cut points). We simulated trials of 280 patients total with no censoring, and all patients followed to failure. On the basis of 10,000 replications, the power was approximately 90%. A total of 280 total patients with 25% benefiting from the new treatment corresponds to about 70 patients benefiting. We found in chapter 4 that for an enrichment design in which the hazard ratio was 0.5, about 72 events are required for 90% power with a one-sided 5% significance level. Consequently, the adaptive threshold design evaluated in this situation had about the same statistical power as the enrichment design, although the appropriate cut point was not known in advance. The two calculations are not entirely commensurate, however, because our simulation took advantage of the known exponential distribution. Also, the power estimated here by simulation used the null distribution computed by simulating trials under a simple null hypothesis and that may somewhat overestimate the power compared to using the permutation significance test. Nevertheless, it appears that the adaptive threshold design enabled an appropriate threshold to be determined efficiently. Hence, having a limited number of candidate cut points does not appear to substantially impair the ability to identify a treatment effect limited to a marker-based subset of patients utilizing the approach described here. Further evaluations of the power of the adaptive threshold design are warranted however.

7

Multiple Predictive Biomarkers

Predictive Analysis of Clinical Trials

In this chapter, we consider the situation in which one is planning a clinical trial comparing a new treatment to a control but does not have a single predictive biomarker identified at the start of the trial. We consider two situations: one in which a small set of candidate markers is identified before starting the trial and the other in which many markers are being measured.

7.1 Designs Based on Few Candidate Biomarkers

We first consider the situation in which a relatively small (e.g., ≤ 5) set of candidate predictive biomarkers are available for use in a phase III clinical trial evaluating a new treatment E relative to a control C, and we are interested in identifying a single marker that identifies patients for whom the new treatment is superior to control. Each marker may either be binary or ordered with multiple candidate cut points. We assume that there are M candidate markers and K_j candidate cut points $b_1^j, \ldots, b_{K_j}^j$ for marker j. The permutation significance test described in Chapter 6 for the adaptive threshold design is easily extended to this more general situation. Let l_k^j denote the log likelihood of the data under an assumption that there is no treatment effect for patients with marker j less than or equal to b_k^j and a common treatment effect for patients with marker j greater than b_k^j. For each marker j, we compute the log likelihood maximized over the possible cut points

$$l_{\max}^j = \max \left\{ l_1^j, l_2^j, \ldots, l_{K_j}^j \right\}. \tag{7.1}$$

We then maximize over the biomarkers to obtain the test statistic

$$\max \left\{ l^1_{\max}, l^2_{\max}, \ldots, l^M_{\max} \right\}. \tag{7.2}$$

The null distribution of (7.2) is approximated by permuting the treatment labels, recalculating the l^j_k values for all biomarkers j and all cut points j, and then recalculating the maximum (7.2). This process is repeated for a thousand or more permutations of the treatment labels, and the 95th percentile of the maximum values is selected as the critical value for the test. If the value of (7.2) for the actual treatment labels is beyond that critical value for the null permutation distribution, then the null hypothesis is of no benefit, for the new treatment is rejected.

This approach is recommended if the number of candidate biomarkers is not large. When the number of candidates is too large, the distribution of the test statistic under the null hypothesis is so broad that the statistical power is poor for identifying treatment effects and the methods described later in this chapter are more appropriate.

If the global null hypothesis is rejected at the 5% level, then the next step is to identify which of the candidate biomarkers are most useful and to develop an indication classifier that identifies the range of biomarker values that renders a patient a good candidate for the new treatment. If the global null hypothesis is rejected, then a permutation significance test based on (7.1) can be performed for each individual test at the 5% level to determine which tests individually identify patients who benefit from the new treatment. These M individual tests can each be performed at the 5% level because the initial test based on (7.2) protected the study-wise type I error to be no greater than 5%. The individual tests are performed to provide guidance in the selection of useful biomarkers. For each individual test that is statistically significant, a probabilistic indication classifier can be developed using either the bootstrap confidence interval approach or the Bayesian approach described in Chapter 6.

Utilizing multiple candidate biomarkers has implications for sample size planning. Statistical power will depend on the number of candidate biomarkers, the number of candidate thresholds per biomarker, the distributions of the individual biomarkers and the correlations among them, and the alternative hypothesis. All these characteristics except the last can be estimated from archived specimens. The permutation test based on (7.2) automatically adjusts for correlations among the biomarkers. When there are five biomarkers that are highly correlated, then the null distribution of the test statistic (7.2) will be very similar to the null distribution for a single biomarker. When the markers are weakly correlated, the null distribution is broader.

Sample size planning for this approach can be carried out using a simulation approach. For example, one would specify the number of candidate markers, the candidate cut points for those markers, and the correlation between the markers. One would examine hypotheses in which outcomes for all patients come from a specified null distribution F_0, except for patients on the new treatment with marker value above a specified cut point of one of the specified candidates. For those patients, outcomes are drawn from an alternative distribution F_1. For each sample size to be evaluated, one can generate multiple sets of data based on this specification. For each set of clinical trial data simulated, statistical significance of the result is determined by performing the permutation test described earlier. A sample size is selected that provides adequate power for the alternative hypothesis of interest.

When there is a single prespecified cut point for each candidate biomarker, a simpler conservative approach to sample size planning is possible. Let p_i denote the p value for comparing treatments within the set S_i of patients having biomarker i above the prespecified cutoff. Then one can conservatively claim a treatment effect if $\min\{p_i\} \leq 0.05/M$, where M is the number of candidate markers. Suppose that there are five candidate markers and each has a cut point defined with only 25% of the patients having positive values. As for the example of enrichment design in Chapter 4, we may wish to have 90% power for detecting a halving of the hazard for this subset of patients. This was seen to require 72 events in the test-positive patients when the significance test was performed at a 0.05 one-sided level. In the discussion of stratification design in Chapter 6, we suggested splitting the 0.05 between a test of overall treatment effect and a test restricted to the marker-positive subset. Here we will just assume that one of the markers is a dummy marker that counts all patients as positive. With $M = 5$, including the dummy marker, the significance test should be conducted at the $0.05/5 = 0.01$ level. This is conservative for treatment planning purposes because it does not take into account the correlation among the tests. The 72 events computed with a significance level of 0.05 becomes 109 events for a significance level of 0.01. Because only 25% patients are assumed marker positive, the clinical trial would be sized to observe a total of $4 * 109 = 436$ events.

7.2 Designs for Development and Validation of Multivariate Classifiers

The design described in the previous section is for settings with a small number of candidate biomarkers. In that circumstance, it is possible to optimize classifier development over the individual candidates using the full sample and properly adjust for the optimization process. When there is a large number of candidates or when the classifiers of interest include those utilizing combinations of the candidates, then the development and validation processess are more complex. In these circumstances, there are so many possible classifiers based on combinations of the candidate variables that even under the null hypothesis of uniform treatment ineffectiveness, many classifiers will appear to identify a responsive subset of patients. Consequently, special methods of model development must be used that are sensitive to avoiding model overfitting. Also, some form of sample splitting or cross-validation must be used to separate model development from evaluation of treatment effects in the subsets determined by the model. We will discuss such designs after describing some examples of predictive classifiers.

7.2.1 Predictive Classifiers

A predictive classifier is a function that identifies the patients who appear to benefit from the new treatment E compared to the control C. A pre-specified algorithmic analysis plan is applied to a data set D to generate a "predictive classifier" $F(\underline{x};D)$, where $\underline{x}$ denotes the vector of variables available. This vector may include candidate biomarkers of a priori interest or may include variables with no a priori credentials for predictive classification.

$F(\underline{x};D) = 1$ means that a patient with covariate vector $\underline{x}$ is predicted to benefit from receiving E rather than C, whereas $F(\underline{x};D) = 0$ indicates that patient is not predicted to benefit from E. This is a predictive classifier based on comparing two treatment groups, not the more familiar kind of prognostic classifier for a single group. This classifier is developed based on analyzing outcome and covariates for the two treatment groups in the training set. Freidlin and Simon (2005) developed a weighted voting-predictive classifier based on genes whose expression levels indicate an interaction with treatment in predicting outcome. Many other types of classifier development algorithms are possible, and the design can be used broadly, not just when the covariates represent gene expression measurements. For example, with survival data, one could use a proportional hazards model

$$\log \frac{h(t; \underline{x}, z)}{h_0(t)} = \alpha z + \underline{\beta}' \underline{x} + z \underline{\eta}' \underline{x} \tag{7.3}$$

where z is a treatment indicator $z = 0$ for C and $z = 1$ for E, and where $\underline{x}$ denotes the vector of covariates. This model can be fit on the training set in a variety of ways. For example, one can use a supervised principal components approach, as follows (Bair and Tibshirani 2004). One first screens the variables $x_1, \ldots, x_p$ one by one by examining the significance of the variable by treatment interaction in models containing only one of the candidate variables; that is, for each candidate variable $x_1, \ldots, x_p$, one fits the model

$$\log \frac{h(t; x_i, z)}{h_0(t)} = \alpha z + \beta_i x_i + z \gamma_i x_i \tag{7.4}$$

and evaluates the significance of the interaction regression coefficient γ_i. One then selects the variables in which the interactions are significant at a prespecified significance level and computes the first principal component of the selected variables. The first principal component is a weighted average of these selected variables with the weights $w_1, \ldots, w_p$ determined to maximize the variance subject to the restriction that the squares of the weights must sum to 1. For this supervised principal component approach, only the variables selected as having significant interactions are allowed to have nonzero weights. For a patient with vector of covariates $\underline{x}$, let $u(\underline{x}) = \sum_i w_i x_i$ denote the value of the first principal component. The model used for survival prediction is

$$\log \frac{h(t; u(\underline{x}), z)}{h_0(t)} = \alpha z + \beta u(\underline{x}) + z \gamma u(\underline{x}). \tag{7.5}$$

This is a proportional hazards model involving only a single covariate, that being the first supervised principal component. The effects of the multiple variables are combined into a single variable.

For the model (7.5), the difference in log hazard for a patient with covariate vector $\underline{x}$ receiving treatment E ($z = 1$) compared to that same patient receiving treatment C ($z = 0$) is

$$\delta(\underline{x}) = \alpha + \gamma u(\underline{x}).$$

This treatment effect can be estimated by $\hat{\delta}(\underline{x}) = \hat{\alpha} + \hat{\gamma} u(\underline{x})$, where $\hat{\alpha}$ and $\hat{\gamma}$ are the estimated regression coefficients obtained by fitting model (7.5) on the training set.

This $\hat{\delta}$ function can be used to predict whether future patients are likely to benefit from the new treatment more than the control. Patients with the most negative values of $\delta(\underline{x})$ are predicted to be the most likely to benefit from E relative to C. To classify patients in the validation set, a cut point must be defined. This can be a predetermined value such as zero, a predetermined quantile of the values of $\delta(\underline{x})$ in the training set can be used, or the cut point can be optimized as a tuning parameter. All tuning parameters should be optimized by cross-validation within the training set.

An alternative classifier can be based on a generalization of the compound covariate method of Radmacher, McShane, and Simon (2002, 86). The prognostic compound covariate is defined by

$$v_1(\underline{x}) = \sum_i \frac{\hat{\beta}_i}{\text{ser}(\hat{\beta}_i)} x_i$$

where the summation is over the variables with regression coefficients β_i significant at a prespecified significance level in the univariate models (7.4). Similarly, the predictive compound covariate is defined by

$$v_2(\underline{x}) = \sum_i \frac{\hat{\gamma}_i}{\text{ser}(\hat{\gamma}_i)} x_i.$$

Prediction is based on the proportional hazards model involving only treatment and the two compound covariates (Matsui et al. 2012):

$$\log \frac{h(t; \underline{x}, z)}{h_0(t)} = \alpha z + \beta^* v_1(\underline{x}) + z\eta^* v_2(\underline{x}). \tag{7.6}$$

For classifying a future patient with covariate vector $\underline{x}$ using (7.6), the difference in log hazard for a patient with compound covariate values $(v_1(\underline{x}), v_2(\underline{x}))$ receiving treatment E compared to that same patient receiving treatment C is estimated as $\hat{\alpha} + \hat{\eta}^* v_2$. This function can be used to classify or rank patients in the validation set. Patients with the most negative values of $\hat{\alpha} + \hat{\eta}^* v_2$ are predicted to be the most likely to benefit from E relative to C. For evaluating prediction accuracy, one would classify patients in the validation set into quantiles based on their values of $\hat{\alpha} + \hat{\eta}^* v_2$ and examine the actual treatment effect within those quantiles by computing Kaplan-Meier curves for each treatment, with separate pairs of curves for the different quantiles.

7.2.2 Probabilistic Predictive Classifier

If there are few enough candidate biomarkers that they all can be included in the proportional hazards model (7.3), then a probabilistic predictive classifier can be developed in the following manner. The difference in log hazard for a patient treated with E and the same patient treated with C is $\hat{\delta}(\underline{x}) = \hat{\alpha} + \hat{\underline{\eta}}'(\underline{x})$. This is an estimate because it is dependent on the training set T. For large training sets, this estimate is normally distributed with mean $\delta(\underline{x}) = \alpha + \underline{\eta}'\underline{x}$ and variance estimated as $\sigma^2(\underline{x}) = (1, \underline{x})'\Sigma(1, \underline{x})$, where Σ denotes the covariance matrix associated with the estimated $(\hat{\alpha}, \hat{\eta})$ parameters. A reasonable decision rule for determining whether to use the new treatment E or the control C might be to use E if the true $\delta(\underline{x}) \leq \Delta$ and use C otherwise, where the cut point Δ is prespecified based on the toxicity and cost difference between the treatments. The reason for the less than or equal sign is that a negative value of $\delta(\underline{x})$ means that the hazard for E is less than the hazard for C. This true classifier cannot be used because the true $\delta(\underline{x})$ is not known; however, because the distribution of $\hat{\delta}(\underline{x})$ is known, we can develop a probabilistic classifier as follows:

$$\Pr[E\,\text{preferred for patient}] = \Pr[\delta(\underline{x}) \leq \Delta]$$

$$= \Phi\left\{ \frac{\Delta - \left(\hat{\alpha} + \hat{\underline{\eta}}'\underline{x}\right)}{\sqrt{\left(1, \hat{\underline{\eta}}\right)' \Sigma \left(1, \hat{\underline{\eta}}\right)}} \right\} \qquad (7.7)$$

where Φ denotes the cumulative distribution function of the standard normal distribution. This derivation is informal but can be rigorously justified in a frequentist manner.

Expression (7.7) cannot be used as a probabilistic classifier in high-dimensional settings when variable selection is used in estimation of the regression coefficients. In that case, the assumption of normality for the parameter vector is no longer correct.

7.2.3 Adaptive Signature Design

Freidlin and Simon (2005, 307) published an adaptive signature design for using genome-wide gene expression profiling to develop and evaluate a predictive classifier in a phase III clinical trial. Their design is, however, broadly applicable to any set of biomarkers that can be used in combination to define a predictive classifier. (Simon, 2012 in press).

At the time of final analysis, one starts by comparing outcomes for the experimental treatment group E to the control group C for all randomized patients. If this overall treatment effect is not significant at a reduced level α_1, the full set P of patients in the clinical trial is partitioned into training set T and validation set V. A prespecified algorithmic analysis plan is applied to the training set to generate a predictive classifier $F(\underline{x}, T)$, where $\underline{x}$ denotes the vector of variables available. This vector may include candidate classifiers or variables with no a priori credentials for predictive classification.

Once a single completely specified classifier is defined on the training set, it is used to classify the patients in the validation set. These patients are classified as either sensitive to the new treatment, that is, predicted likely to benefit from the new treatment E relative to C, or not sensitive. Let S denote the set of sensitive patients in the validation set; that is, $S = \{j \in V \mid F(\underline{x}_j, T) = 1\}$. One then compares outcomes for sensitive patients in the validation set who received E versus sensitive patients in the validation set who received C using a log-rank test.

The adaptive signature design provides a statistically valid framework for including in a single phase III clinical trial both the discovery of a multivariate classifier and the comparison of the treatment arms in the subsets determined by the classifier. The approach seems so simple that it is easy to miss recognizing that it provides a paradigm dramatically different from and superior to standard subset analysis. As widely practiced in clinical trials, standard subset analysis is no more than a large number of statistical significance tests. If the tests to be performed are not defined in advance, then no adjustment for multiplicity is possible. Even when the subsets to be examined are defined in advance, trialists rarely reserve any of the overall type I error of the trial for the subset analysis. Standard subset analysis is often data driven, and no effort is made to obtain unbiased estimates of the treatment effect within subsets.

The adaptive signature approach involves several fundamental principles. These principles may be given insufficient attention by statisticians more interested in the details of developing new types of models. But it is the principles that are most important, not the details of the modeling. One of the principles is that rather than perform a large number of statistical significance tests, the focus is on developing a single predictive classifier. Only one statistical significance test is performed: the test of the treatment effect in classifier positive patients. The approach also provides an unbiased estimate of the treatment effect in classifier-positive patients. A second principle is that if the trial involves a traditional overall test of average treatment effect in all patients, then some of the 5% type I error for the trial must be reserved for the single significance test of treatment effect in classifier-positive patients. The third key principle is that the data used for development of the classifier are separated from the data used for comparing the treatment arms in the classifier-positive subset.

In addition to these key principles, there are many details to be decided in using the adaptive signature design – important details such as what classifier development algorithm to use, what proportion of the sample to use for model development, how to perform the partition into training and validation sets, how to size the trial, and so on. The paper by Sher et al. (2011, 844) describes an example of utilization of the adaptive signature design framework in the evaluation of treatments for castrate-resistant prostate cancer. That publication was developed at a workshop of the Brookings Institution and Friends of Cancer Research to foster collaboration between industry, the U.S. Food and Drug Administration (FDA), and academic oncology to advance the development of improved treatments and the panel presenting the design for that application included FDA representatives.

For the application of the adaptive signature design described by Sher et al. (2011, 844), the overall 0.05 type I error was partitioned into 0.01 for the overall analysis and 0.04 for the comparison of treatments in classifier-positive patients. This was because the power was most constrained for the evaluation of treatment effect in the subset of the validation set. A sample size that provided sufficient power for that subset analysis at the 0.04 significance level provided more than enough patients for the overall analysis at the 0.01 level. The trial design developed had 90% power to detect a reduction in hazard of 25% overall and 80% power for detecting a 45% reduction in hazard for a classifier positive subset that had prevalence of only 33%. Of course, at the start of the trial, one does not know the prevalence of classifier-positive patients because the classifier has not yet been defined. The design developed by Sher et al. devoted 33% of the sample to the training set. Unfortunately, little research has been done on sample size requirements for development of predictive classifiers. Dobbin and Simon (2007, 281) and Dobbin, Zhao, and Simon (2008, 559) studied sample size requirements for development of prognostic classifiers and found that the requirements are somewhat less than one might expect. Their interpretation was that good prognostic classifiers are based on variables whose means are substantially different between the classes. Variables with less different means may be found statistically significant with sufficient sample size, but they are not useful for classification of individual patients. Because large sample sizes are not required to identify variables whose means in the two groups are substantially different, and because many prognostic models for high-dimensional classification are based on the univariate contribution of the component variables (to avoid overfitting), it takes smaller samples than one might expect to develop good prognostic classifiers, if such classifiers exist based on the data available. Similar results, however, have not been shown for development of predictive classifiers.

7.2.4 Cross-Validated Adaptive Signature Design – Predictive Analysis of Clinical Trials

Freidlin, Jiang, and Simon (2010) demonstrated that the statistical power of the adaptive signature design can be substantially increased by embedding the classifier development and validation process in a K-fold cross-validation rather than using a single training set – validation set split. This idea is very powerful and much more broadly applicable than in the context described by Freidlin, Jiang, and Simon (2010) as discussed by Simon (2012, in press).

In the cross-validated adaptive signature design, it is essential to prospectively define an algorithm A for classifying patients as likely or not likely to have better outcome on the new treatment E compared to the control C. This algorithm constitutes the entire preplanned subset analysis. In contrast to the usual subset analysis, which results in a bunch of statements about statistical significance of treatment effects within multiple subsets, this algorithm results in a single completely determined predictive classifier. The predictive classifier partitions the space of covariate vectors into a region for patients who are predicted to benefit from the new treatment E and a complementary region for patients who are not predicted to benefit from E. Some examples of classifier development algorithms are described in Section 7.2.1. The algorithm A when applied to a data set P defines a completely specified predictive classifier $F(\underline{x}|P)$.

The classifier that will potentially be used in the future is the one obtained by applying the algorithm to the full data set P, that is, $F(\underline{x}|P)$. To evaluate the performance to be expected using the algorithm $F(\underline{x}|P)$ in the future, it is necessary to evaluate the algorithm using cross-validation. It should be emphasized that the cross-validation procedure does not provide some abstract characteristic of the algorithm A; it provides an estimate of the predictive accuracy of the classifier $F(\underline{x}|P)$ obtained by applying A to the full set of data P.

The cross-validation is performed in the following way. The full set (P) of patients in the clinical trial is partitioned into K disjoint subsets $P_1, \ldots, P_K$. The ith training set T_i consists of the full set of patients, except for the ith subset, that is, $T_i = P - P_i$. Let $F(\underline{x}|T_i)$ denote the binary classifier developed by applying the algorithm A to training set T_i. Use this classifier to classify the patients in the omitted subset P_i. Let $v_j = F(x_j|T_i)$ denote the predictive classification for patients j in P_i; $v_j = 1$ if the patient is predicted to be sensitive to the new treatment E relative to control C, and zero otherwise. Since the patients in P_i were not included in the training set T_i used to train $F(x|T_i)$, this classification is predictive, not just evaluating goodness of fit to the same data used to develop the classifier. Because each patient appears in exactly one P_i, each patient is classified exactly once, and that classification is done with a classifier developed using a training set not containing that patient.

Let S denote the set of patients j for whom $v_j = 1$, that is, patients who are predicted to be sensitive to the new treatment. We can evaluate the treatment effect expected in the future for patients classified as sensitive to the new treatment using the full sample classifier $F(x|P)$ by comparing outcomes of the patients in S who received treatment E to the outcomes for the patients in S who received the control C. The treatment effect for future patients who are classifier positive using $F(x|P)$ is a random variable because the data set P is a sample of all the possible data sets that could have been used for developing the classifier. The mean value of that treatment effect is estimated by the empirical treatment effect for patients in the subset S of P determined by cross-validation.

Let $L(S)$ denote a measure of difference in outcomes between patients in S who received E and those in S who received C. For example, one could use a log-rank statistic if outcomes are time to event. We can generate an approximation to the null distribution of L by repeating the entire cross-validation analysis for thousands of random permutations of the treatment labels. This test can be used as the primary significance test of the clinical trial to test the global null hypothesis that the new treatment and control are equivalent for all patients on the primary end-point of the trial. Alternatively, it can be used as a fallback test as described for the adaptive signature design.

Having rejected the global null hypothesis described earlier, the application of the algorithm A to the full data set P provides an indication classifier decision support tool $F(x|P)$ that can be used to inform labeling of the new treatment or by physicians for informing treatment decisions for their patients. The classifier recommended for future use is the one obtained by applying the algorithm to the full data set, that is, $F(x;P)$. The K-fold cross-validation provides a proper estimate of treatment effect for the subset who are predicted to benefit using this full sample classifier. Freidlin, Jiang, and Simon (2010) showed that the hazard ratio for E versus C in the cross-validated set S is a conservative estimate of the hazard ratio for the sensitive set of the full sample classifier, that is, for the set of future patients with covariate vectors for which $F(\underline{x}|P) = 1$.

The effectiveness of the indication classifier based on $F(x|P)$ depends on the algorithm used. Algorithms that overfit the data will provide classifiers that make poor predictions, and the expected outcomes may be substantially worse than using the traditional approach. Algorithms based on Bayesian models with many parameters and noninformative priors may be as prone to overfitting as frequentist models with many parameters. The effectiveness of an algorithm will also depend on the data set, that is, the unknown truth about how treatment effect varies among patient subsets. A strong advantage of the proposed approach, however, is that an almost unbiased estimate of the performance of a defined algorithm can be obtained from the data set of a clinical trial itself. This is clearly preferable to performing exploratory analysis on the full data set without any cross-validation, reporting the misleading fit of the model to the same data used to develop the model and cautioning that the results need testing in future clinical trials.

The approach described here can also be used in a clinical trial for which the overall average treatment effect is significant. The approach permits one to identify, based on covariate profiles, the patients who do and do not benefit from the new treatment. Rather than just focusing on the patients predicted to be sensitive to the new treatment, one also compares treatment effects for the complementary subset defined by the cross-validated classifications. To illustrate this, we have applied this predictive analysis of clinical trials to data from the gene expression profiling study conducted on pretreatment biopsy specimens from 181 patients with diffuse large-B-cell lymphoma (DLBCL) who received a standard chemotherapy combination called CHOP, and 233 patients with this disease who received R-CHOP (CHOP plus the antibody rituximab) (Lenz et al., 2008, 827). Unfortunately, this was not a randomized clinical trial, but the data will serve to illustrate the method of analysis.

These data were analyzed using the cross-validated predictive analysis described above with Dr. Jyothi Subramanian (Simon, in press, 845). The only clinical covariate considered for this analysis was the international prognostic index (IPI). For the purpose of this analysis, the IPI was categorized into two groups – subjects with IPI scores of 0, 1, or 2 were categorized as "low," and subjects with IPI scores of 3, 4, or 5 were called "high." For some of the subjects, one or more of the variables that make up the IPI were missing. If, for a given subject, the value for the missing variable would not change the IPI group call (e.g., depending on the value of the missing variable, the IPI value would be either 1 or 2), then the subject would be included as a member of that IPI group. However, if the missing value could make a difference (e.g., between 2 and 3), then that subject was excluded from our analysis. Thirty-nine subjects were excluded because the IPI group could not be determined. Of the resulting 375 subjects, 262 fell in IPI class "low," and 113 subjects were in IPI class "high." The end-point was overall survival (death from any cause). Prior to the start of analysis, one subject with a survival time of zero was removed, resulting in 374 subjects for this analysis.

Gene expression and clinical data were obtained from the Gene Expression Omnibus (acc. no. GSE10846). To account for the differences in microarray preprocessing between R-CHOP and CHOP samples, the expression values for each gene in the R-CHOP group were adjusted so that their medians matched the median of the CHOP group (21). For the predictive analysis, the data were log2 transformed, and the 1,000 genes with the highest variance were used.

A Cox proportional hazards (ph) regression model was developed using patients in both CHOP and R-CHOP groups. A 10-fold cross-validation was applied to estimate predictive accuracy. Univariate gene selection was used as the feature selection method. For each gene, a Cox proportional hazards model was developed in the training set using treatment, covariate (IPI), gene, and treatment by covariate and treatment by gene interactions. Ten genes with the lowest p values for the treatment by gene interactions were selected for inclusion in the multivariate Cox ph model. The multivariate Cox model was again developed using treatment, IPI, 10 best genes, treatment by IPI, and treatment by gene interactions. Gene selection and multivariate model development were all done within each cross-validation loop. In the multivariate Cox model, let $\hat{\delta}$ be the estimated main effect of treatment and $\hat{\gamma}$ be the estimated vector of interaction coefficients. Then, for a patient in the test set with vector $\underline{x}$ of covariates corresponding to the variables of the predictive model developed in the corresponding test set, $F(\underline{x}) = 1$ if $\hat{\delta} + \hat{\gamma}'\underline{x} \leq c$ where c was fixed to be the median of the $F()$ values in the corresponding training set.

Figure 7.1 shows the results of the overall analysis. The results of applying the predictive algorithm in a 10-fold cross-validation loop are shown in Figures 7.2 and 7.3. For the sensitive subset of patients who appear to benefit from R-CHOP, the value of the log-rank statistic for the separation of the cross-validated survival curves is 19.67, and the permutation p value is 0.005 (200 permutations). For this sensitive subset, the log hazard ratio is -1.12, and the bootstrap-based 95% confidence interval for the log hazard ratio is $(-1.40, -0.125)$ (200 bootstrap samples). For the complementary subset of patients who do not appear to benefit from R-CHOP, the value of the log-rank statistic for the cross-validated survival curves is 0.81, and the permutation p value is 0.49 (200 permutations). The predictive analysis has thus identified a group of patients who appear unlikely to benefit from R-CHOP.

Related methods for developing individualized estimates of treatment efficacy have been studied by Cai et al. (2011), Foster, Taylor, and Rubery (2011), Rubin and van der Laan (2012), Zhang et al. (2012), and Matsui et al. (2012).

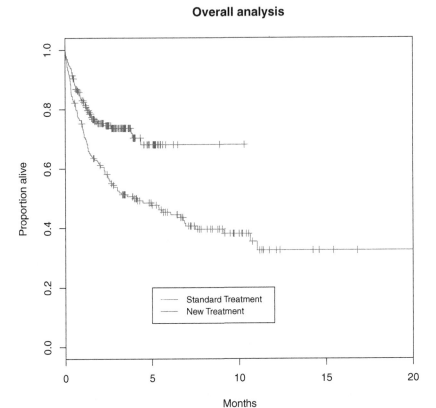

Figure 7.1. Overall analysis. The value of the log-rank statistic is 14.1, and the corresponding *p* value is 0.0002. The new treatment R-CHOP thus shows an overall benefit.

Cases predicted to benefit from new treatment

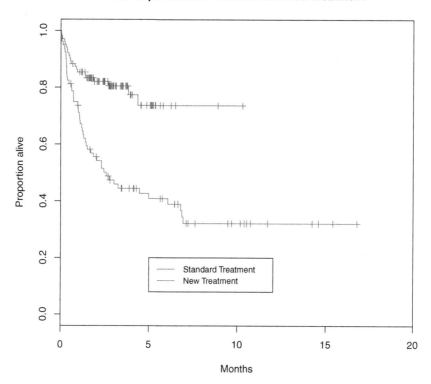

Figure 7.2. Predictive analysis. Cross-validation was used to predict patients who would benefit or not from the new treatment. This figure shows the survival curves for patients predicted to benefit from the new treatment. The value of the log-rank statistic for the separation of the survival curves is 19.67, and the permutation p value is 0.005 (200 permutations). The hazard ratio is -1.12, and the bootstrap-based 95% confidence interval for the hazard ratio is $(-1.40, -0.125)$ (200 bootstrap samples).

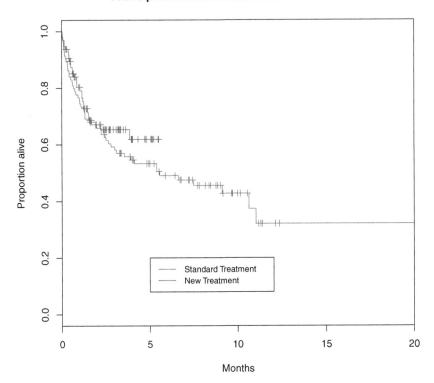

Figure 7.3. Survival curves for cases predicted no benefit from new treatment. The value of the log-rank statistic in this case is 0.81, and the permutation p value is 0.49 (200 permutations).

8

Prospective–Retrospective Design

Sometimes, a new candidate predictive biomarker is identified after the definitive trials have demonstrated benefit for the specific drug, making new prospective randomized clinical trials of that agent impractical. Simon et al. (2009) indicated that in some cases, it may be possible to use archived specimens collected in the past from appropriate, previously conducted therapeutic trials in a way that preserves the focus, control of type I error, and statistical power of properly designed fully prospective studies. Indeed, when there is substantial preliminary evidence that a new marker predicts benefit from a specific drug, it may sometimes be possible to assay the marker in archived specimens from randomized clinical trials that were conducted to evaluate the drug, as was done for KRAS mutations in colorectal cancer (Amado et al., 2008, 591; Karapetis et al., 2008, 671).

When suitable archived tissue is available, this prospective–retrospective approach can facilitate and expedite delivery of valuable cancer diagnostics that may be of considerable benefit to patients. Simon et al. (2009) developed stringent conditions required for such a prospective–retrospective approach to have a degree of reliability that approaches that of a fully prospective clinical trial, and proposed a refinement to the previously published Level of Evidence (LOE) Scale that permits a more critical analysis of the quality of tumor marker studies using archived specimens.

Although biomedical scientists and biostatisticians are taught that prospective studies are good and retrospective studies are bad, the distinction between prospective and retrospective is often confused with the distinction between experimental and observational. For studies of prognostic and predictive biomarkers in oncology, the term *retrospective* is in some cases misleading. In cancer epidemiology, both retrospective case control studies and prospective cohort studies are observational, rather than experimental, studies. Neither type of study involves random assignment of exposure, and hence, observed correlations between exposures and disease do not provide as strong a basis for claims of causality as in experimental studies. The most serious limitation of epidemiologic studies is their nonexperimental nature, not whether they are retrospective or prospective.

In therapeutics, many retrospective analyses are also nonexperimental, with treatment selection based on patient factors and referral pattern rather than on randomization. Such studies are also often conducted without a written protocol and are unfocused, with numerous patient subsets and end-points compared without control for the overall chance of a false positive conclusion. In contrast, prospective randomized clinical trials contain internal control of treatment assignment, careful and proscribed data collection (including outcomes and endpoints), and a focused analysis plan that is developed before the data are examined.

Many biomarker studies are conducted with convenience samples of available specimens, which are assayed for the marker with no prospectively determined subject eligibility, power calculations, marker cut point specifications, or analytical plans. Such studies are likely to result in highly biased conclusions. However, if a retrospective study is designed to use archived specimens from a previously conducted prospective trial, and if certain conditions are prospectively delineated in a written protocol before the marker study is performed, Simon et al. (2009) asserted that it might be better termed a prospective–retrospective study. Such a study should carry considerably more weight toward determination of clinical utility of the marker. Having multiple studies of different candidate biomarkers based on archived tissues from the same prospective trial would, however, present a greater opportunity for false positive conclusions than a single fully prospective trial focused on a specific biomarker. Consequently, independent confirmation of findings for a specific biomarker in multiple prospective–retrospective studies is important.

Important considerations in the design of a reliable prospective–retrospective study include (1) the use of an assay analytically validated for use with archived specimens; (2) the use of archived specimens from clinical trials with appropriate design and sample size to address the utility of a specific intended clinical use of the marker; (3) a written completely specified analysis plan for the biomarker analysis focused on a single maker, ideally with a prespecified cut point for marker positivity; (4) adequate proportion of patients in the clinical trials with archived specimens available and demonstration that sample availability is independent of treatment assignment within the clinical trial; and (5) results that are verified, or validated, in more than one clinical trial.

To apply the prospective–retrospective approach, the investigator should have a clear idea of the specific intended use for the assay. In general, this will be as a prognostic factor to identify patients with sufficiently good prognosis on standard therapy that they do not require a more intensive approach, or as a predictive factor to determine whether a particular type of therapy is likely to be effective. To establish medical utility of a prognostic marker, a randomized trial is sometimes not necessary, as noted at the end of Chapter 2. For example, a prospective single-arm trial in which chemotherapy is withheld from patients at a low risk of recurrence is used in the portion of the TAILORx clinical trial designed to validate the very favorable prognostic outcomes in the low recurrence score population. Assuming that preanalytical (tissue handling) factors are well controlled and match current practice activities, and that the clinical data are collected in a fashion typical of a clinical trial, archived tissue from a sufficiently large population of untreated patients may be adequate to permit accurate estimates of recurrence based on tumor marker subgroups for determination of clinical utility of the marker.

Tumor response data from a single-arm phase II clinical trial of a specified treatment can be used to establish the clinical validity of a biomarker for predicting response to that treatment, but a larger randomized trial with a survival or progression-free survival end-point is generally required to establish the medical utility of the predictive marker.

8.1 Levels of Evidence

In the original American Society of Clinical Oncology (ASCO) LOE Scale, retrospective studies were determined to be in category II or worse (Hayes et al., 1996, 333). Simon et al. (2009) proposed an updated revision of the LOE Scale, in which more precise definitions are provided for the types of studies that might be used to analyze the clinical utility of a biomarker and in which retrospective studies using archived specimens might reach level I evidence. The level of evidence for the medical utility of a biomarker relates to key factors involving patients, specimens, assays, and statistical analysis plans.

In the original LOE Scale, level I evidence of medical utility of a biomarker required a prospective clinical trial. Patients are entered, treated, and followed prospectively according to a prewritten protocol; the study is prospectively powered specifically to address the tumor marker question; and specimens are collected, processed, and assayed for the marker in real time. The prospective trial will generally not utilize a marker strategy design, as described at the end of Chapter 2, however, because of the serious limitations of that design. Compelling results from one such prospective trial would be considered definitive, and no other validating trial would be required. This strategy was included in the original level of evidence scale proposed by ASCO as LOE I and continues to be their gold standard.

In the revised LOE Scale, a second strategy to obtain level I evidence would be to perform a prospective-retrospective tumor marker study using archived specimens from a prospective trial that addresses a therapeutic question and accommodates the current marker question. As indicated earlier, to evaluate a predictive marker, the prospective trial would generally need to be a randomized trial that compares the treatment with an appropriate control treatment. Patients are prospectively enrolled, treated, and followed, and specimens are prospectively collected, processed, and archived using generic standard operating procedures. The tumor marker question might be identified during the conduct of the trial or after its completion, but the specification of the tumor marker hypothesis should be based on data completely external to the trial. In fact, tissues archived from the trial should not be assayed until a new protocol has been written that focuses on the evaluation of the specified marker with a completely specified statistical analysis plan. Prior to undertaking the study, the assay should be analytically and preanalytically validated for use with archived tissue, and the assay should be performed blinded to the clinical data. Because the trial was designed to address the therapeutic question, it will often be underpowered to establish the statistical significance of treatment by marker interaction (Peterson & George, 1993, 418). It may, however, be adequately sized to reliably identify a large treatment effect restricted to test-positive patients, as might be expected for a predictive biomarker. Nevertheless, even with these caveats, results from such a study will be more likely to arise from chance than from a fully prospective approach.

It is clearly desirable that the available specimens from the archived bank should be representative of the patients who were accrued to the study as a whole, although there is no guarantee that the study patients are themselves representative of the general population of patients. Although there is no minimal requirement that can be universally applicable, Simon et al. (2009) suggest that the correlative study should include at least two-thirds of the total accrued cases or that they be selected in a fashion that strives to avoid selection bias.

For the prospective–retrospective approach to be sufficient to change practice, Simon et al. (2009) required that the results must be confirmed using specimens from a second study based on archived tissue from a different trial that has been designed, conducted, and analyzed in a similar, if not identical, manner. The results of these two studies must be consistent and compelling to change clinical practice. Furthermore, these validation studies need to be performed using the same assay or similar assays that clearly identify the same marker.

Ideally, any new medical intervention will be adopted into clinical practice only in the setting of level I evidence, and ideally, such evidence is generated in a prospective randomized clinical trial. However, such trials are not always feasible. In the case of tumor markers, practice guidelines and the availability of other diagnostic procedures can sometimes make it very difficult to perform new clinical trials because such trials may involve withholding of therapy that is considered standard of care. Even when they are considered ethical, such trials usually require many years to conduct and are quite expensive. For new drug development, in many cases, an analytically validated companion diagnostic test will not be available, or the appropriate biological measurement may not be clear at the time that the pivotal trials of the drug are initiated, as for the use of KRAS mutation as a predictive biomarker for anti-EGFR antibodies in colorectal cancer (Amado et al., 2008, 591; Karapetis et al., 2008, 671; Allegra et al., 2009, 669).

Archived tissue specimens from high-quality clinical trials can therefore be of great importance for establishing the medical utility of a prognostic or predictive biomarker. For such an evaluation to be more useful than just for generating hypotheses, we summarize the following necessary conditions:

1. Archived tissue adequate for a successful assay should be available on a sufficiently large number of patients from the pivotal trials to permit appropriately powered analyses and to ensure that the patients included in the biomarker evaluation are clearly representative of the patients in the pivotal trials.
2. Substantial data on analytical validity of the test should exist that ensure that results obtained from the archived specimens will closely resemble those that would have been obtained from analysis of specimens collected in real time. Assays should be conducted blinded to the clinical data.
3. The analysis plan for the biomarker evaluation should be completely developed prior to the performance of the biomarker assays. Both the analysis plan for the biomarker study and the design of the trial(s) whose samples were selected for analysis should be appropriate for the evaluation of a companion diagnostic had it been undertaken at the outset. The analysis should be focused on a single, completely defined diagnostic classifier. For multigene classifiers, the mathematical form of combining the individual components, weights, and cut points should be specified beforehand. In general, the analysis should not be

exploratory, and practices that might lead to a false positive conclusion should be avoided.

4. The results should be validated in at least one or more similarly designed studies using the same assay techniques.

Statistics Background

In this appendix, we provide a brief review or introduction to some of the basic statistical concepts used in the chapters.

A.1 Statistical Significance

We will introduce the concept of statistical significance of treatment effects using the permutational approach. Suppose we have outcome data from n patients in a control group C and n patients in the experimental treatment group E. We want to test the null hypothesis that the experimental treatment is equivalent to the control in its effect on outcome. Let T denote a measure of difference between the outcomes on the experimental treatment and the outcomes on the control. With outcomes like blood pressure, we might define T as the mean outcome for patients on E minus the mean for those on C. With continuous outcome measures, the difference in mean outcomes is often standardized by the within-group standard deviation. If the outcome is a binary measure of response or no response, then T might be the difference between the treatment and control groups in the proportion responding.

If the null hypothesis were true, the outcomes would be the same whether patients were treated by E or C. This is called the global null hypothesis and is the one that we will consider. Let N denote the total number of patients. The N treatment assignments can be collected into a vector. The ith element of the vector is E if the ith patient to enter the clinical trial was assigned E; otherwise, the ith element is C. There are many other treatment assignment vectors that could have resulted from the randomization process. Let's let S denote the set of randomization vectors that could have resulted. For each of the alternative randomization vectors, the outcomes of all the patients are unchanged if the null hypothesis is true. For each of these alternative randomization vectors, however, the mean outcome of the patients who would have received E and the mean outcome of those who would have received C do change compared to what they were in the actual study because the patients who would have received E and the patients who would have received C change.

Generally there are an enormous number of alternative randomization vectors, but suppose we examine a random m of them denoted by $i = 1, 2, \ldots, m$. We might take m to be 1,000 or even 10,000. For each of these randomization vectors, we recompute the mean outcome for patients who would have been on E minus the mean outcome of patients who would have been on C. Call these values $T_1, T_2, \ldots, T_m$. These m values describe the null distribution of our test statistic (difference in means) that we expect to see under the null hypothesis. If the treatment E is really effective in lowering blood pressure, we expect that the T statistic for the actual data should be smaller than most of the $T_1, T_2, \ldots, T_m$ values that we would see if the null hypothesis were true. In fact, the one-sided statistical significance level is defined as the proportion of the $T_1, T_2, \ldots, T_m$ that are less than or equal to T for the actual data. That is, if $m = 1,000$ and five of those values computed for alternative randomization vectors are less than or equal to the T value for the real data, then the one-sided significance level is 5/1,000 or 0.005. In this situation, the two-sided significance level is taken as twice the one-sided value to account for the fact that the absolute value of the difference in means could be small if the mean for patients on E is much lower than the mean for patients on T, or vice versa.

The test described above is called a permutation test. Permutation tests are driven directly by the null hypothesis and randomization process and are not based on assumptions about the shape of the distribution of the outcome data. In some cases, for large sample sizes, the distribution of the test statistic under randomly sampled permutations has a known form, and statistical significance can be computed without randomly generating the permutations. We have described the permutation test in the simplest situation, with a single outcome per patient and no covariates. Permutation tests are applicable to more complicated settings, however. The commonly used nonparametric tests like the Mann–Whitney test are permutation tests in which the test statistic is based on the ranks of the observations. Permutation tests are commonly used even in settings without experimental randomization.

Many commonly used statistical significance tests are derived based on an assumed population sampling model rather than a permutation model. For example, a t test for the situation considered earlier assumes that the outcomes for patients treated with the new treatment E have a normal distribution with unknown mean μ_E and unknown variance σ^2 and the outcomes for patients treated with the control regimen C have a normal distribution with unknown mean μ_C and the same variance σ^2. If we have a random sample of n patients from each of the two distributions and wish to test the null hypothesis that $\mu_E = \mu_C$, then we can base that test on the sample means $\bar{y}_E$ and $\bar{y}_C$ and variances s_E^2 and s_C^2 for the experimental and control groups. The test statistic is the difference in sample means divided by the standard error of that difference:

$$t = \frac{\bar{y}_E - \bar{y}_C}{\hat{\sigma}\sqrt{2/n}}$$

where $\hat{\sigma}^2 = (1/2)\left(s_E^2 + s_C^2\right)$ is the pooled estimate of the unknown common variance. The factor of $2/n$ in the denominator of the t statistic reflects the fact that the variance of a sample mean based on n observations equals the variance of the individual observations divided by n and that the variance of the difference of independent sample means equals the sum of the variances of the sample means. The standard error of the difference of two sample means is just the square root of the variance of the difference of the means. If the numbers of observations in the two groups were unequal, then the formula for the t statistic and the formula for the pooled variance would be slightly modified. If the null hypothesis is true, then the t statistic shown above should have a standard t distribution with $2n - 2$ "degrees of freedom." To do the significance test, one would compute the t statistic and refer to the table of the t distribution with $2n - 2$ degrees of freedom to find the area of the tail beyond the value of the computed t. That is the p value, or significance level, of the test. The t test is less intuitive than the permutation test because it assumes that the distribution of outcomes for all eligible patients who would receive each of the two treatments E and C has a Gaussian (i.e., normal) form, that the variances are equal, and that we have sampled randomly from those hypothetical populations. In fact, randomizing treatment assignment does not mean that we are randomly sampling patients from a target population.

A.2 Confidence Interval

An important feature of the population sampling framework is that it enables us to compute confidence limits for the unknown difference in true population means $\mu_E - \mu_C$. From the assumption of normality, it can be shown that

$$\Pr \left[t_{\alpha/2} \leq \frac{\left(\bar{y}_E - \bar{y}_C\right) - \left(\mu_E - \mu_C\right)}{\hat{\sigma}\sqrt{2/n}} \leq -t_{\alpha/2} \right] = 1 - \alpha$$

where $t_{\alpha/2}$ is the $100\,(\alpha/2)$ percentile of the t distribution with $2n - 2$ degrees of freedom. This can be rearranged to the form

$$\Pr \left[\left(\bar{y}_E - \bar{y}_C\right) + t_{\alpha/2}\hat{\sigma}\sqrt{2/n} \leq \left(\mu_E - \mu_C\right) \leq \left(\bar{y}_E - \bar{y}_C\right) \right.$$
$$\left. - t_{\alpha/2}\hat{\sigma}\sqrt{2/n} \right] = 1 - \alpha.$$

This provides a confidence interval for the unknown difference $\mu_E - \mu_C$ because the upper limit and lower limit can be computed. For example, if $\alpha = 0.05$, then one has 95% confidence that the unknown difference is between the upper limit and lower limit. In interpreting the meaning of this confidence limit, it is useful to remember that the unknown means are regarded as fixed but unknown numbers. Because we have a limited sample of patients, the sample means and the sample standard deviations are subject to variation. Consequently, the upper and lower limits are random and variable. The confidence limit means that the probability that these two limits bound the true but unknown difference in means is 95%. Simon (1986, 466) provided a review of confidence intervals for treatment effects in clinical trials with various types of end-points.

A.3 Statistical Power

Statistical power is the probability of rejecting the null hypothesis that there is no difference in the true unknown means for the two treatments. The power depends on the true difference in the distributions of outcomes of the two treatments, on the sample size, and on the level of statistical significance desired. Consider the circumstance described above with a continuous outcome y. Assume that y is normally distributed with means μ_E and μ_C for the two treatment groups and common variance σ^2. For simplicity, assume that the common variance is known. The null hypothesis that $\mu_E = \mu_C$ is rejected if the difference in sample means $\bar{y}_E - \bar{y}_C$ divided by the standard error of the difference is beyond the upper tail point of the normal distribution corresponding to the statistical significance level. This can be written

$$\Pr[\text{reject } H_0] = \Pr[\bar{y}_E - \bar{y}_C > k_{1-\alpha}\sigma\sqrt{2/n}]$$

because the standard error of the difference in sample means is the standard deviation σ of individual measurements times the square root of 2 divided by the sample size of n patients per treatment arm. Using the fact that the difference in sample means is normally distributed with mean $\mu_E - \mu_E$ and standard deviation $\sigma\sqrt{2/n}$, the probability of rejecting the null hypothesis can be written

$$\begin{aligned}
\Pr[\text{reject } H_0] &= \Pr\left[\frac{(\bar{y}_E - \bar{y}_C) - (\mu_E - \mu_C)}{\sigma\sqrt{2/n}} > k_{1-\alpha} - \frac{(\mu_E - \mu_C)}{\sigma\sqrt{2/n}}\right] \\
&= \Phi\left\{\frac{(\mu_E - \mu_C)}{\sigma\sqrt{2/n}} - k_{1-\alpha}\right\}
\end{aligned}$$

where Φ denotes the cumulative distribution function of the standardized normal distribution with mean 0 and standard deviation 1. If we want the power to equal a prespecified quantity $1 - \beta$, then the argument of Φ must equal $k_{1-\beta}$, the $100(1 - \beta)$th percentile of the standardized normal distribution. Consequently,

$$n = 2\frac{(k_{1-\alpha} + k_{1-\beta})^2}{\left(\dfrac{\mu_E - \mu_C}{\sigma}\right)^2}. \qquad (A.1)$$

This formula gives the sample size per treatment arm needed to have power $1 - \beta$ for achieving a one-sided statistical significance level α. The denominator on the right-hand side of the equation is the standardized treatment effect, that is, the difference in means expressed relative to the standard deviation of individual observations. The sample size is critically dependent on the reciprocal of the square of this standardized treatment effect. Similar expressions can be developed for sample size planning with binary response or survival end-points.

A.4 Survival Data

Survival data are an example of "right-censored" data. That means that the survival time is known for some patients, but for patients still alive at last follow-up, we only know that the survival time will be at least as great as that observed. Because of the right-censored nature of survival data, special methods of statistical analysis are needed. Survival data are often represented by estimating the survival distribution $S(t)$, which is defined as the probability that survival is greater than or equal to t for all values of t. The standard method of estimating $S(t)$ is the Kaplan–Meier method (Kaplan & Meier, 1958, 351), which is reviewed in Marubini and Valsecchi (1995, 391). There are two other functions that can be derived from $S(t)$. One is the survival density function, which is the time derivative of $S(t)$, denoted by $S'(t)$. The negative of the survival density can be thought of as the instantaneous rate of failure. The other function is the hazard function, which is the instantaneous rate of failure at t conditional on having survived up to t. The hazard function can be expressed as $- S'(t)/S(t)$.

Many useful methods for the analysis of survival data are based on the proportional hazards model. This model was introduced by Cox

(1972, 848) and elucidated by Kalbfleisch and Prentice (2002, 849). The Mantel–Haenszel test (Mantel, 1963, 852) and log-rank test (Peto, Pike, & Armitage, 1977, 422) are significance tests for comparing survival distributions, and sample size planning is based on a model in which it is assumed that the ratio of hazard functions for the two distributions is constant over time. These tests are based on an estimate of the hazard ratio. Let $\hat{\delta}$ denote the logarithm of this estimate. Under the null hypothesis, $\hat{\delta}$ is approximately normally distributed with mean 0 and variance $4/D$, where D denotes the total number of events. By a derivation similar to that leading to (A.1), to have statistical power $1 - \beta$ for rejecting the null hypothesis at a one-sided significance level of α when the true log hazard is δ, the number of total events required is approximately

$$D = 4\frac{\left(k_{1-\alpha} + k_{1-\beta}\right)^2}{\delta^2}. \tag{A.2}$$

For an accessible introduction to the analysis of survival data, see Marubini and Valsecchi (1995, 391).

A.5 Linear Regression

Many statistical analyses are based on a regression model rather than using a permutation test. For example, if the outcome is a quantitative measurement such as blood pressure, then a normal linear regression model might be used:

$$E(y) = \alpha + \beta_1 x_1 + \beta_2 x_2 + \cdots + \beta_p x_p \tag{A.3}$$

which indicates that the expected value of the outcome variable y depends on the value of p variables $x_1, x_2, \ldots, x_p$. The unknown regression coefficients $\beta_1, \beta_2, \ldots, \beta_p$ determine the relative contributions of the variables, and there is an intercept α. In clinical trials, the variable x_1 might be defined as equal to 1 if the patient receives treatment E and 0 if the patient is in the control group. The other variables $x_2, \ldots, x_p$ may be prognostic covariates that are also thought to potentially influence outcome.

With linear regression, the estimates $\hat{\alpha}, \hat{\beta}_1, \ldots, \hat{\beta}_p$ of the unknown parameters are determined to minimize the sum of squares of differences between the observed outcome values $y_1, \ldots, y_n$ for the n patients and the predicted values

$$\hat{y}_i = \hat{\alpha} + \hat{\beta}_1 x_{i1} + \hat{\beta} x_{i2} + \cdots + \hat{\beta} x_{ip}. \tag{A.4}$$

The sum of squares can be written

$$\sum_{i=1}^{n} \left(y_i - \left(\hat{\alpha} + \hat{\beta}_1 x_{i1} + \hat{\beta} x_{i2} + \cdots + \hat{\beta} x_{ip} \right) \right)^2. \tag{A.5}$$

The least squares approach is a special case of the method of maximum likelihood for estimating the parameters for regression models. When the outcome variables are normally distributed with means described by (A.1) and common variances denoted by σ^2, the likelihood of outcome y_i is

$$\left(\frac{1}{\sqrt{2\pi}\sigma} \exp \left\{ -\frac{\left(y_i - \left(\alpha + \beta_1 x_{i1} + \beta_2 x_{i2} + \ldots + \beta_p x_{ip} \right) \right)^2}{2\sigma^2} \right\} \right). \tag{A.6}$$

The likelihood function for this normal regression is the product of the factors described in (A.6) over all the cases $i = 1, 2, \ldots, n$. The likelihood function represents the probability of obtaining the data observed as a function of the parameters. If one takes the natural logarithm of that likelihood function, the likelihood function reduces to the negative of form shown in (A.5) plus some terms that do not involve the unknown regression parameters. Hence, for normal linear regression, the estimated parameters that minimize the sum of squared differences between the observed and predicted outcome values are the estimates that maximize the likelihood function.

A.6 Logistic Regression

For binary outcome data or survival data, the normal linear regression model of (A.3) is no longer appropriate because the outcome y is binary and the linear regression equation does not reflect that. For binary outcome data, the logistic regression model shown here is generally used instead of (A.1):

$$\log\left(\frac{p}{1-p}\right) = \alpha + \beta_1 x_1 + \beta_2 x_2 + \cdots + \beta_p x_p \qquad (A.7)$$

where p denotes the probability of a response and log denotes natural logarithm. Expression (A.7) implies that

$$p = \frac{\exp\left(\alpha + \beta_1 x_1 + \beta_2 x_2 + \cdots + \beta_p x_p\right)}{1 + \exp(\alpha + \beta_1 x_1 + \beta_2 x_2 + \cdots + \beta_p x_p)}$$

$$1 - p = \frac{1}{1 + \exp\left(\alpha + \beta_1 x_1 + \beta_2 x_2 + \cdots + \beta_p x_p\right)}$$

for the probability of response ($y = 1$) and the probability of failure ($y = 0$), respectively. The method of maximum likelihood is still used for estimating parameters. The likelihood factor for a patient with outcome y_i is p if $y_i = 1$ and $1 - p$ if $y_i = 0$. The full likelihood function is thus

$$\prod_{i=1}^{n} \left\{ \frac{\exp\left(\alpha + \beta_1 x_{i1} + \beta_2 x_{i2} + \cdots + \beta_p x_{ip}\right)}{1 + \exp(\alpha + \beta_1 x_{i1} + \beta_2 x_{i2} + \cdots + \beta_p x_{ip})} \right\}^{y_i}$$

$$\cdot \left\{ \frac{1}{1 + \exp\left(\alpha + \beta_1 x_{i1} + \beta_2 x_{i2} + \cdots + \beta_p x_{ip}\right)} \right\}^{1-y_i} .$$

The logarithm of this function can be maximized to obtain the estimates $\hat{\alpha}, \hat{\beta}_1, \ldots, \hat{\beta}_p$. As the sample size n becomes very large, these estimates can be approximated by a multivariate normal distribution with mean vector being the true values of the regression coefficients. The covariance matrix of the maximum likelihood estimators can be estimated from the inverse of the matrix of second derivatives of the log likelihood function evaluated at the maximum likelihood estimates. For more details, see Cox and Snell (1989, 850).

A.7 Proportional Hazards Regression

When the outcome data consist of survival times or disease-free survival times, the proportional hazards model is usually used instead of the linear regression model (A.3) or the logistic model (A.7). The value of the hazard function at time t of a survival distribution is the probability of failure immediately following t conditional on survival up to t. The proportional hazards model assumes that the hazard function can be factored into the product of a function of t that does not involve the covariates and a function of the covariates that does not involve time:

$$h(t, x_1, x_2, \ldots, x_p) = h_0(t) \exp\left(\alpha + \beta_1 x_1 + \beta_2 x_2 + \cdots + \beta_p x_p\right). \quad (A.8)$$

The reason that this model is so popular is that the regression coefficients can be estimated without specifying $h_0(t)$. The likelihood function, called the partial likelihood, can be written

$$\prod_{i=1}^{n} \delta_i \frac{\exp\left(\alpha + \beta_1 x_{i1} + \beta_2 x_{i2} + \cdots + \beta_p x_{ip}\right)}{\sum_{j:t_j \geq t_i} \exp\left(\alpha + \beta_1 x_{j1} + \beta_2 x_{j2} + \cdots + \beta_p x_{jp}\right)} \quad (A.9)$$

where t_i denotes the survival time of the ith patient and the censoring indicator δ_i equals 1 for a failure and 0 if the survival time is censored. The partial likelihood is a product over patients whose survival times are not censored. For such a patient i, the numerator is the hazard function for the ith patient and the denominator is the sum of the hazard functions for all patients who are still alive at time t_i. Because of the separability of the hazard function, the $h_0(t_i)$ factors cancel out of the numerator and denominator factors. As with logistic regression, the estimates of the regression coefficients are obtained by maximizing the logarithm of (A.9). These estimates are approximately multivariate normal for large sample sizes, and the covariance function can be estimated as described for logistic regression. For more details, see Kalbfleisch and Prentice (2002, 849).

The regression methods described above can be used for studying the effects of candidate prognostic factors on outcome. The book by Harrel (2001, 853) provides a comprehensive approach for such modeling. For such modeling, the candidate prognostic factors should all be specified in advance and should be included in the regression model. The regression model, with the maximum likelihood estimates plugged in for the values of the regression coefficients, can be used for predicting outcome for new patients. In addition to a maximum likelihood estimate of each regression coefficient, one also obtains an approximate standard error of the estimate. Since the maximum likelihood estimates are approximately normal for large samples, one can test the null hypothesis that a regression coefficient is zero. This is a test of whether that regression coefficient is zero in the context of the other covariates being included in the model. Unfortunately, the validity of these statistical results depends on all the covariates being specified in advance and being included in the model. Any use of the data for variable selection to optimize the fit or the simplicity of the model invalidates these statistical significance results. Regression modeling is often used in an informal way. The variable selection often practiced may give a misleadingly optimistic view of the fit of the model to the data or of the importance of some variables.

Regression modeling is also often used to evaluate a treatment effect while controlling for prognostic factors. As mentioned previously, we might model x_1 as a binary (0 or 1) indicator of treatment C or E and include the other variables thought to be prognostic. It is even more important in this setting that the prognostic covariates be specified in advance and that no data-dependent variable selection be used in the modeling. Under these circumstances, if the sample size is sufficient, then the maximum likelihood estimate of the regression coefficient associated with x_1 divided by the estimated standard error of that estimate can be used to compute the significance of the treatment effect after adjustment for the effects of the other variables. There are other ways of adjustment for covariates in evaluating a treatment effect in a clinical trial, but regression methods provide a general framework.

A.8 Bayesian Methods

The statistical methods described previously are called *frequentist* because they regard probabilities as reflecting the frequency of summary statistics computed on data. The data are regarded as random selections from fixed but unknown distributions. One makes inferences about the parameters of the unknown distributions based on the observed statistics. The frequentist methods are distinguished from Bayesian methods, in which probabilities are often regarded as reflecting subjective individual beliefs about the values of the parameters of the unknown distributions. For example, in the discussion of the t test given earlier, the true mean values of the outcome distributions μ_E and μ_C were regarded as unknown fixed values. A Bayesian approach, however, would regard μ_E and μ_C as values for which we have probability distributions that represent our belief in their possible values.

Before performing the clinical trial, our probability distributions for μ_E and μ_C are called *prior distributions.* Bayes's theorem tells us how to update our prior distributions after observing the data to obtain our *posterior distributions* for μ_E and μ_C. Suppose that the prior probability that μ_E and μ_C take on values (x, y) is $f(x,y)$. Let D_E and D_C denote the data for the experimental and control treatments, respectively. The likelihood function can be thought of as the probability of getting data D_E and D_C. That probability depends on the true values μ_E and μ_C. Let $L(\mu_E, \mu_C)$ denote this likelihood function. Bayes's theorem indicates that the posterior probability that μ_E and μ_C take on values (x, y) is

$$f(x, y | D_E, D_C) = kL(x, y) f(x, y).$$

The left-hand side is the posterior probability that the means are x and y, respectively, given (the vertical bar) that the data D_E and D_C have been observed. The k on the right-hand side is just a normalizing constant that is determined to ensure that the left-hand side integrates to 1 over the range of all possible (x, y) pair values.

Bayesian methods are flexible because a prespecified experimental design is not necessary for computing posterior probabilities. Bayesian statistics provides a way of representing our personal view of uncertainty about unknown quantities. These measures of uncertainty can then be used for decision making. There is a formal theory of decision making under uncertainty that uses the Bayesian paradigm (Berger, 2010, 846). To employ the approach, one must define a personal loss function reflecting the relative loss one would suffer if one took action A and the true values of the unknown means were μ_E and μ_C, denoted $G(A; \mu_E, \mu_C)$. The expected loss is thus the expected value of the loss with regard to the posterior distribution of μ_E and μ_C, that is,

$$\int G(A; \mu_E, \mu_C) f(x, y | D_E, D_C) d\mu_E d\mu_C$$

where the integral is over the range of possible values of the unknown means. With a pure Bayesian approach, the concept of type I error is not of intrinsic importance.

Bayesian methods are flexible and can be useful for decision-making settings in which a subjective prior distribution can be elicited that actually reflects personal prior uncertainty about the unknown parameters. Bayesian methods are less generally useful in phase III clinical trials because the personal priors of the trialists may be of no relevance to the broad community of consumers of the results of the clinical trial. The prior distributions of trialists influence actions such as how large to make the trial and when to terminate the trial, and the posterior distributions reflect both the prior distributions and the data; hence those with different prior distributions may find the conclusions of the trialists unconvincing. In certain circumstances, prior distributions can be formulated for some parameters that would be broadly acceptable to a broad community (Spiegelhalter & Freedman, 1994, 508). Bayesian methods are also sometimes employed for phase III trials using noninformative prior distributions with interim monitoring rules and decision regions that ensure that the type I error does not exceed 5%. This approach is primarily a frequentist approach, however, with test statistics and monitoring regions motivated by Bayesian considerations. So-called noninformative priors in many cases do not reflect our usual prior belief that small mean differences are more likely than large mean differences. Many extensive discussions of the Bayesian approach are available (e.g., Rubin, 2009, 847).

Prognostic Classifiers Based on High-Dimensional Data

Good studies, whether prospective or retrospective, whether involving a single protein, genome-wide gene expression profiling, or DNA sequence analysis, require clear goals and careful planning if they are to be successful. Planning is driven by experimental objectives. Unfortunately, many prognostic factor studies and studies involving DNA microarray experiments do not have clear objectives and are not successful. Here, however, we will emphasize clear objectives and careful planning. We are not attempting to provide here a thorough description of the analysis of DNA microarray data. For that see texts such as that by Speed (2003) or Simon, Korn, McShane et al. (2004). One type of objective commonly encountered in DNA microarray experiments is identification of variables (e.g., genes) differentially expressed among predefined classes of samples. We will refer to this as the class comparison objective. A related but distinct objective that is more relevant to the topic of this book is development of a mathematical function that can accurately predict the prognosis of a patient based on measured variables. This will be referred to as class prediction or prognostic classification. Most research on prediction with high-dimensional data is focused on class prediction when there are two classes. We review some of the methodology available for this case and then discuss its extension to prognostic classification when the outcome is survival or some other right-censored time-to-event variable.

Before discussing class prediction, first let us distinguish it from *class discovery*. Class discovery is fundamentally different than class comparison or class prediction in that no classes are predefined. Usually class discovery is for the purpose of determining whether discrete subsets of a disease entity can be defined based on the gene expression profiles. This is different from determining whether the expression profiles correlate in some way with some already known diagnostic classification. Cluster analysis of one type or another is used for class discovery but is not effective for class prediction.

Cluster analysis refers to an extensive body of methods of partitioning samples into groups based on the pair-wise distances or similarities of the measured variables. Cluster analysis is considered an unsupervised method because class membership indicators are not utilized (or do not exist). The pair-wise distance measures between expression profiles are generally computed with regard to the complete set of genes represented on the array which are well measured with sufficiently high signal strength, or all the genes that show meaningful variation across the set of samples. Even if the classes do group into clusters based on an unsupervised distance metric, the analysis does not provide a useful class predictor that can be validated on an independent sample or used for new cases.

B.1 The Development of Classifiers

In this section we present some of the important aspects of the development and validation of classifiers. For a more complete development, see Hastie, Tibshirani, and Freedman (2009). Let x_i denote the vector of measurements for the ith sample. If the data are from a gene expression microarray, the vector may contain the logarithm of the signal value that summarizes the background-adjusted intensity values for all of the probes or probe sets on the array. Logarithmic transformation of the signal values is often recommended because the range of values is typically very large for single-label arrays. For dual-label arrays, the components of the x_i vector will usually be the logarithm of the ratio of the background-adjusted intensity of the label for the experimental sample relative to the label of the common reference sample. The candidate predictor variables could alternatively be binary indicators of the somatic mutation status of each gene or categorical indicators of the polymorphic status of each SNP from a genotype of the germ line of the patient.

For class prediction, associated with each sample i is a class label c_i. For problems with two classes, we may think of the labels as being 0 and 1, but the particular encoding used is generally not important. A class predictor is a mathematical function that takes an input vector x and produces a class label c. A mathematical function is merely a mapping from one set (the set of all predictor vectors x) to another set (the set of class labels). It does not have to have a simple algebraic form.

The most important requirement for a class predictor is that it predict accurately. Neils Bohr supposedly once said, "Prediction is difficult, particularly the future." But it is the future that we want to predict. We do not really care about predicting the class of the samples available to us now. We want to be able to predict class membership for future samples whose class membership we do not know. The current samples are available to enable us to develop a predictor function and to help us estimate how accurate the class predictor we develop will be for future predictions. In using our current samples both to develop a predictive classifier and to estimate its accuracy for future predictions, we will have to be careful to simulate true future prediction. Otherwise, our estimates may be very biased and quite misleading, as discussed later.

For class prediction problems, our objective is to develop a predictor that will give accurate predictions in the future and to provide an estimate of that accuracy. Our objective is not to determine what genes are differentially expressed among the classes. As we have defined it, determining which genes are differentially expressed is the objective of class comparison, not of class prediction. In the process of developing a class predictor, we will generally select genes to include in our predictor, but the objective of this gene selection is to develop an accurate predictor. The way we do gene selection may be quite different when our objective is accurate prediction compared to when our objective is to make inferences about which genes are differentially expressed. This distinction is often missed.

B.2 Components of Class Prediction

Although we have defined a class predictor as a function that maps an input vector x to a class label c, most class predictors do not use all the components of the input vector. Consequently, one part of developing a class predictor is determining which variables to include in the predictor. This is generally called *feature selection* or, in the context of microarray prediction, *gene selection*.

It is well known from the theory of linear regression that including too many noise variables in the predictor reduces the accuracy of prediction. A noise variable is a variable that is not related to the quantity being predicted. Feature selection is particularly important in high-dimensional prediction because the number of noise variables may be orders of magnitude greater than the number of relevant variables. The influence of the genes that actually distinguish the classes may be lost among the noise of the more numerous noise genes unless we select the informative genes to be utilized by the class predictor.

The second main component of a class predictor is specification of the mathematical function that will provide a predicted class label for any given input vector x. There are many kinds of predictor functions, such as diagonal linear discriminant analysis, nearest, neighbor predictors, support vector machines, and decision trees.

Most kinds of predictors have parameters that must be assigned values before the predictor is fully specified and able to provide specific predictions. These parameters are in many ways equivalent to the regression coefficients of ordinary linear regression. The machine learning literature calls the process of specifying the parameters "training." Predictive functions often contain tuning parameters. These might include a parameter that determines the number of variables (genes) to include in the model and a cut point for transforming a numerical predictive score into a classification. Completely specifying the predictor means specifying the type of predictor, the genes included, and the values of all parameters, including tuning parameters.

B.3 Estimating the Accuracy of a Class Predictor

How can we develop a proper estimate of the accuracy of class prediction for future cases? For a future case with vector x of variables, we will apply a fully specified predictor developed using the data available today. The most satisfactory approach is to have separate validation dataset for evaluating the predictive accuracy of the classifier of interest. This "external validation" approach can better reflect the variety of sources of variation for future samples than can internal validation approaches (Taylor, Ankerst, & Andridge 2008). If we are to emulate the future predictive setting in developing our estimate of predictive accuracy and do not have a separate validation dataset, we must set aside some of our samples and make them completely inaccessible until we have a fully specified predictor that has been developed without utilizing any of those set-aside samples.

To properly estimate the accuracy of a predictor for future samples, the current set of samples must be partitioned into a training set and a separate test set. The test set emulates the set of future samples for which class labels are to be predicted. Consequently, the test samples cannot be used in any way for the development of the prediction model. This means that the test samples cannot be used for estimating the parameters of the model, and they cannot be used for selecting the genes to be used in the model. It is this later point that is often overlooked.

Rosenwald et al. (2002, 80) used this split-sample approach successfully in their international study of prognostic prediction for large-cell lymphoma. They used two-thirds of their samples as a training set. Multiple kinds of predictors were studied on the training set. When the collaborators of that study agreed on a fully specified prediction model, they accessed the test set for the first time. On the test set, there was no adjustment of the model or fitting of parameters. They merely used the samples in the test set to evaluate the predictions of only one model; one that was completely specified using only the training data.

Cross-validation is an alternative to the split sample method of estimating prediction accuracy. There are several forms of cross-validation (Molinaro & Simon, 2005, 396). Here we will describe *leave-one-out cross-validation* (LOOCV). LOOCV starts like split-sample cross-validation in forming a training set of samples and a test set. With LOOCV, however, the test set consists of only a single sample; the rest of the samples are placed in the training set. The sample in the test set is placed aside and not utilized at all in the development of the class prediction model. Using only the training set, the informative genes are selected, and the parameters of the model are fit to the data. Let us call M_1 the model developed with sample 1 in the test set. When this model is fully developed, it is used to predict the class of sample 1. This prediction is made using the expression profile of sample 1 but obviously without using knowledge of the true class of sample 1. Symbolically, if $\underline{x}_1$ denotes the complete expression profile of sample 1, then we apply model M_1 to $\underline{x}_1$ to obtain a predicted class $\hat{c}_1$. This predicted class is compared to the true class label c_1 of sample 1. If they disagree, then the prediction is in error. Then a new training set–test set partition is created. This time, sample 2 is placed in the test set, and all the other samples, including sample 1, are placed in the training set. A new model is constructed from scratch using the samples in the new training set. Call this model M_2. Model M_2 will generally not contain the same genes as model M_1. Although the same algorithm for gene selection and parameter estimation is used, since model M_2 is constructed from scratch on the new training set, it will in general not contain exactly the same gene set as M_1. After creating M_2, it is applied to the expression profile $\underline{x}_2$ of the sample in the new test set to obtain a predicted class $\hat{c}_2$. If this predicted class does not agree with the true class label c_2 of the second sample, then the prediction is in error.

The process described in the previous paragraph is repeated n times, where n is the number of biologically independent samples. Each time it is applied, a different sample is used to form the single-sample test set. During the n steps, n different models are created, and each one is used to predict the class of the omitted sample. The prediction errors are totaled, and that is the leave-one-out cross-validated estimate of the prediction error.

At the end of the LOOCV procedure, you have constructed n different models. They were only constructed to estimate the prediction error associated with the type of model constructed. The model that would be used for future predictions is one constructed using all n samples. That is the best model for future prediction and the one that should be reported in the publication. The cross-validated error rate is an estimate of the error rate to be expected in use of this model for future samples. This assumes, however, that the relationship between class and expression profile is the same for future samples as for the currently available samples.

A commonly used, but very biased, estimate is called the *resubstitution estimate*. You use all the samples to develop a model M. Then you predict the class of each sample i using its expression profile $\underline{x}_i$; $\hat{c}_i = M(\underline{x}_i)$. The predicted class labels are compared to the true class labels, and the errors are totaled. Radmacher et al. (2002) and Simon et al. (2003, 85) reported on a simulation to examine the bias in estimated error rates for class prediction (see their supplemental information for a full description of the simulation). Two types of LOOCV were studied: one with removal of the left-out specimen prior to selection of differentially expressed genes and one with removal of the left-out specimen prior to computation of gene weights and the prediction rule but after gene selection. They also computed the resubstitution estimate of the error rate. In a simulated data set, 20 gene expression profiles of length 6,000 were randomly generated from the same distribution. Ten profiles were arbitrarily assigned to class 1 and the other 10 were assigned to class 2, creating an artificial separation of the profiles into two classes. Since no true underlying difference exists between the two classes, class prediction will perform no better than a random guess for future biologically independent samples. Hence, the estimated error rates for simulated data sets should be centered around 0.5 (i.e., 10 misclassifications out of 20).

Figure B.1 shows the observed number of misclassifications resulting from each level of cross-validation for 2,000 simulated data sets. It is well known that the resubstitution estimate of error is biased for small data sets, and the simulation confirms this, with an astounding 98.2% of the simulated data sets resulting in zero misclassifications, even though no true underlying difference exists between the two groups. Moreover, the maximum number of misclassified profiles using the resubstitution method was only one.

Cross-validating the prediction rule after selection of differentially expressed genes from the full data set does little to correct the bias of the resubstitution estimator: 90.2% of simulated data sets still result in zero misclassifications. It is not until gene selection is also subjected to cross-validation that we observe results in line with our expectations: the

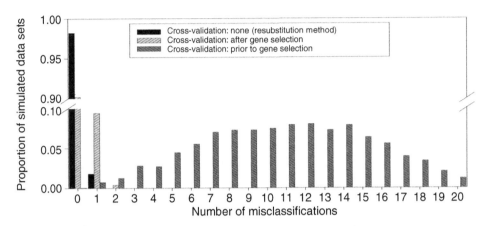

Figure B.1. The effect of various levels of cross-validation on the estimated error rate for prediction with random data.

median number of misclassified profiles jumps to 11, although the range is large (0–20). The simulation results underscore the importance of cross-validating all steps of predictor construction in estimating the error rate. Nevertheless, Dupuy and Simon (2007, 285) and Subramanian and Simon (2010a) have documented how frequently the misleading resubstitution estimate is reported in publications in major medical journals.

B.4 Class Prediction Algorithms

Many algorithms have been used successfully for class prediction, for a more comprehensive review of algorithms, see Hastie, Tibshirani, and Friedman (2009) or Dudoit, Fridyland, and Speed (2009). Some class prediction problems are quite easy. For example, distinguishing tumors that originate from different cell types is generally easy if the cell types are quite different because different types of cells may have hundreds or thousands of genes that are differentially expressed. Problems of this type, therefore, are not generally an adequate test of a class prediction algorithm. One problem with many publications is that they demonstrate a new algorithm using a relatively easy problem and fail to demonstrate that the new method performs better than standard algorithms for the same sets of data.

For many class prediction problems, the key is identifying a set of genes that are individually differentially expressed among the classes. This is called feature selection. Simple classification algorithms based on good features are effective for many class prediction problems.

B.4.1 Feature Selection

The most commonly used approach to feature selection is to identify the variables that have different means in the classes when considered individually. For example, if there are two classes, one can compute a t test or a Mann–Whitney test for each variable. The variables that are significantly differentially expressed at a specified significance level are selected for inclusion in the class predictor. The stringency of the significance level used controls the number of variables that are included in the model. If one wants a class predictor based on a small number of genes, the threshold significance level is made very small. Issues of multiple testing or false positives are not really relevant, however, because the objective is only to select features for inclusion in the model; no particular claim is made about the selected genes. Similarly, it does not matter whether the assumptions of the t test are strictly satisfied because the p values are merely used as a convenient index for selecting genes. Some methods do not use p values at all but merely select the m most differentially expressed genes and specify m arbitrarily. The class means of some genes that are significantly differentially expressed between two classes may not be large. Such genes are often not useful for class prediction of individual cases. The significance level depends on the difference in means divided by the standard error of the difference. For a large sample size, this ratio may be large although the difference in means between the classes is small. This is because the standard error of a mean is the standard deviation of an individual measurement divided by the square root of the number of cases in the class. Prediction accuracy, however, depends on the difference in means divided by the standard deviation of individual measurements, not divided by the standard error. Although the standard errors may be small enough for the difference in class means to be significant, if the difference in class means is not large, assay variability may be too great for accurate diagnosis of individuals. Hence, it is often useful to restrict feature selection to select variables with substantial differences in class means or class means divided by the standard deviation of individual measurements.

Several authors have developed methods to identify optimal sets of genes that together provide good discrimination of the classes. Bo and Jonassen (2002, 95) consider the discrimination ability of all pairs of genes and select the pairs that provide the best discrimination in the training set of samples. Ooi and Tan (2003, 97) and Deutsch (2003, 96) use genetic algorithms to try to identify optimal gene sets for classification. There is little evidence, however, that complex methods based on genetic algorithms provide improved predictive performance (Lai, Reinders, & van't Veer et al., 2006). For prediction problems with more variables (p) than cases (n), it is always possible to find a linear classifier that perfectly separates the classes in the training set. There is rarely sufficient data in the training set to guide the fitting of complex nonlinear classifiers.

Some investigators have used linear combinations of gene expression values as predictors (West, Blanchette, & Dressman, 2001, 28; Khan et al., 2001, 87). The principal components are linear combinations that show the greatest variability among the cases and are orthogonal to each other. Using principal components provides a vast reduction in the dimension of the expression data but has two serious limitations. One is that the weights given to each gene in the principal components are based on variation among samples without regard to classes. Hence, the principal components are not necessarily good predictors. Bair and Tibshirani (2004, 191) used *supervised principal components* as predictive variables. These are principal components of those genes with substantial differential expression among the classes. The second problem is that the principal components have weights for all the genes. Consequently, prediction using principal components requires that expression of all the genes be measured. The method of gene shaving attempts to provide linear combinations with properties similar to the principal components but with small weights made zero (Hastie et al., 2000, 331). Partial least squares methods (Nguyen, & Rocke 2002) provide linear combinations that are maximally correlated with the class indicator.

B.4.2 Classifier Types

Many algorithms have been used effectively with DNA microarray data for class prediction. Dudoit and Fridlyand (2003, 157) and Dudoit, Fridlyand, and Speed (2002, 42) compared a wide variety of algorithms using several publicly available data sets. The algorithms compared included several variants of linear discriminant analysis, nearest-neighbor classification, and several variants of classification trees. A linear discriminant is a function

$$l(\underline{x_i}) = \sum_{j \in F} w_j x_{ij}, \tag{B.1}$$

where x_{ij} denotes the value of the jth variable in sample i, w_j is the weight given to that variable, and the summation is over the set F of features (genes) selected for inclusion in the class predictor. For a two-class problem, there is a threshold value d, and a sample with expression profile defined by a vector $\underline{x_i}$ of values is predicted to be in class 1 or class 2, depending on whether $l(\underline{x_i})$ as computed from equation (B.1) is less than the threshold d or greater than d, respectively.

A large number of class predictors are based on linear discriminants of the form shown in (B.1). They differ with regard to how the weights are determined. The oldest form of linear discriminant is Fisher's linear discriminant (Fisher, 1936). To compute these weights, one must estimate the correlation between all pairs of genes that were selected in the feature selection step. The study by Dudoit and Fridlyand (2003, 157) indicated that Fisher linear discriminant analysis did not perform well unless the number of selected genes was small relative to the number of samples. The reason is that in other cases, there are too many correlations to estimate, and the method tends to be unstable and overfit the data.

Diagonal linear discriminant analysis is a special case of Fisher linear discriminant analysis in which it is assumed that there is no correlation among genes. For diagonal linear discriminant analysis, the weights can be expressed as

$$w_j = \frac{\left(\overline{x}_j^{(1)} - \overline{x}_j^{(0)}\right)^2}{v_j} \cdot \text{sign}\left(\overline{x}_j^{(1)} - \overline{x}_j^{(0)}\right) \tag{B.2}$$

which is the squared difference in the class means of variable j divided by the pooled estimate of the intraclass variance of variable j times the sign of the difference in class means.

It is obviously not true that there is no correlation among genes, but by ignoring such correlations, one avoids having to estimate many parameters and obtains a method that often performs better when the number of samples is small. Golub et al.'s (1999, 12) weighted voting method and the compound covariate predictor of Radmacher, McShane, and Simon (2002, 86) are similar to diagonal linear discriminant analysis and tend to perform very well when the number of samples is small. They compute the weights based on the univariate prediction strength of individual genes and ignore correlations among the genes.

Inner product kernel support vector machines do class prediction using a predictor of the form of equation (B.1). The weights are determined by optimizing a misclassification rate criterion, however, instead of a least squares criterion, as in linear discriminant analysis. Although there are more complex forms of support vector machines (SVMs), they do not appear to be superior to inner product kernel SVMs for class prediction with large numbers of genes (Ben-Dor et al., 2000, 91). There is little motivation for using non–inner product SVMs because the classes are almost always separable for high-dimensional $p > n$ classification problems.

In the study of Dudoit and Fridlyand (2003, 157) and Dudoit, Fridlyand, and Speed (2002, 42), the simplest methods, diagonal linear discriminant analysis and nearest neighbor classification, performed as well or better than the more complex methods for most examples. Nearest neighbor classification is defined as follows. It depends on a feature set F of genes selected to be useful for discriminating the classes. It also depends on a distance function $d(\underline{x}, \underline{y})$, which measures the distance between vectors $\underline{x}$ and $\underline{y}$. The distance function utilizes only the genes in the selected set of features F. To classify a sample with expression profile $\underline{x}$, compute $d(\underline{x}, \underline{y})$ for each sample $\underline{y}$ in the training set. The predicted class of the new case $\underline{x}$ is the class of the case in the training set that is closest to $\underline{x}$ with regard to the distance function d.

There are also several widely used variants of nearest neighbor classification. One is k-nearest neighbor classification. For example, with 3-nearest neighbor classification, you find the three cases in the training set that have vectors that are closest to the vector x of the new case. The class that is most represented among these three samples is the predicted class for x.

A second variant is nearest centroid classification. In the training set, determine the set F of features (variables) that are going to be used for the classification, then compute the centroid of each of the classes. The *centroid* of a class is just the vector of mean values of the variables for cases in that class in the training set. Having determined the centroid for each class, one is ready to classify. With two classes, for example, a new case with vector x of variables is classified as class 1 if x is closer to the centroid of class 1 than to the centroid of class 0. Otherwise, the case is classified as class 0.

The popular shrunken centroid classification method of Tibshirani et al. (2002, 105) is a variation of nearest centroid classification. Rather than computing the centroid of a class as the vector of means of the variables for cases in that class, the variable means are first shrunken toward a grand mean for all the classes combined. The degree of shrinkage is controlled by a tuning parameter that is optimized by cross-validation within the training set. It is a clever method that often performs very well. With nearest centroid classification there is no need to preselect the variables to be used for computing the centroids. The optimization of the shrinkage parameter automatically selects the variables to be included in the classification.

Dudoit and Fridlyand (2003, 157) and Dudoit, Fridlyand, and Speed (2002, 42) also studied some more complex methods such as classification trees and aggregated classification trees. These methods did not appear to perform any better than diagonal linear discriminant analysis or nearest neighbor classification for many of the datasets. Ben-Dor et al. (2000) also compared several methods on several public data sets and found that nearest-neighbor classification generally performed as well or better than more complex methods. Although the linear methods described earlier are most natural for two class problems, the nearest neighbor and nearest centroid methods are not limited by the number of classes.

B.5 Probabilistic Class Prediction

The usual deterministic classifiers provide a prediction of the class of a case based on the measured variables. For some cases, the correct class may be more certain than for other cases, however. The cases for a class can be thought of as a point cloud in a high-dimensional space. The boundaries of the point clouds are uncertain and may overlap. Some cases may lie near the boundary, whereas other cases may be in the interior of a region where one case is predominant. For medical decision making, a probabilistic classifier that provides a probability that the case belongs to each class is often more useful than a deterministic classifier. Kim and Simon (2011, 854) studied the methodology for developing and evaluating probabilistic classifiers with high-dimensional data. We will describe here two of the probabilistic classifiers that they studied.

Let $\underline{x}$ denote a p-dimensional feature vector for a case, and let c denote the class indicator (0 or 1) for that case. Given the training data set of n cases, we are interested in accurately predicting $\Pr[c = 1|\underline{x}]$ for a new case with known feature vector $\underline{x}$. The nearest shrunken centroid method (Tibshirani et al., 2002, 105) is a deterministic classifier in which a new case is classified into the class corresponding to the closest shrunken centroid. The centroid of a class is the vector in which the components of each variable are averaged over the cases in that class in the training set. For the shrunken centroid method, these class-specific centroid vectors are shrunken toward each other. The degree of shrinkage is determined by a tuning parameter, which is optimized to minimize the misclassification rate. This shrinkage forces some of the variables to have the same value in both centroids and thus not be used for the classification. Even for the variables that remain informative, the difference in their shrunken means is less than the difference in their unshrunken means, and this can lead to improved classification accuracy. Let us denote the shrunken mean for the jth variable in class k by $\bar{x}_j^{(k)}$. The intraclass variance of the jth variable is estimated by $(s_j + s_0)^2$, where s_j is the pooled class sample standard deviation for the jth variable and s_0 is a positive constant used for stabilization of variance estimates. Although the shrunken centroid method is usually used as a deterministic classifier, Tibshirani et al. (2002, 105) suggest a way of using the shrunken centroids to obtain a predicted probability for each class k. The distribution of the expression vector $\underline{x}$ is regarded as multivariate normal with a mean vector equal to the shrunken centroid for that class. The covariance matrices (Σ) for the two classes are regarded as equal and diagonal with variance elements $(s_j + s_0)^2$. We denote this multivariate normal probability density by $\phi(\underline{x}; \tilde{x}^{(k)}, \Sigma)$. The probability that the new case is in class 1 is taken as

$$\Pr[c = 1 | \underline{x}] = \frac{\phi\left(\underline{x}; \tilde{x}^{(1)}, \Sigma\right) \pi^{(1)}}{\sum\limits_{k=1}^{K} \phi\left(\underline{x}; \tilde{x}^{(k)}, \Sigma\right) \pi^{(k)}}$$

where the summation in the denominator is over all K classes and $\pi^{(k)}$ denotes the prior probability that a case is in class k. This formula is a plug-in approximation to Bayes's formula for $\Pr[c = 1 | \underline{x}]$ based on assuming multivariate normality with a known diagonal covariance matrix and within class mean vectors given by the shrunken means.

Kim and Simon (2011) also evaluated penalized logistic regression models for two class problems. These models use shrinkage techniques in estimating the coefficients of high-dimensional covariates. Penalties are imposed in the estimation step either on sum of absolute values of regression coefficients or on sum of squared coefficients. Penalized logistic regression models predict class probability for a new case as

$$\Pr[c = 1] = \frac{\exp\{\hat{\alpha} + \hat{\beta}' \underline{x}\}}{1 + \exp\{\hat{\alpha} + \hat{\beta}' \underline{x}\}}.$$

The regression coefficients are determined to maximize a penalized likelihood function. The penalty causes shrinkage of the regression coefficients. The degree of shrinkage can be determined by cross-validation to minimize misclassification error. When an L1 penalty (sum of absolute values of the regression coefficients) is used, a parsimonious model can be obtained, with most of the regression coefficients equal to zero.

Kim and Simon (2011) judged probabilistic classifiers based on the extent to which they are "well calibrated" and on their "refinement." *Well calibrated* means that if a person gathers together the cases for which the predicted probability of being class 1 is some specified value of about w, the proportion of those cases that actually are class 1 is w. Calibration is a measure of the validity of the probabilistic classifier. It is easy to develop a probabilistic model, but that does not mean that the probabilities computed are valid for future data. For example, Bayesian models may reflect your personal view of the likelihood that a new case is from class 1, but unless the model is well calibrated, those personal probabilities will not represent reality. Refinement is a measure for distinguishing among well-calibrated classifiers. It measures the ability of the probabilistic classifier to distinguish cases in the different classes. A probabilistic classifier that produces probabilities of 0.5 for all new cases may be well calibrated if half the cases are from class 1 but is not very refined or useful. A well-calibrated classifier that produces predictions closer to 0 or 1 is more refined and useful.

B.6 Survival Risk Prediction

B.6.1 Survival Risk Classifiers

Classifiers for use with survival data have focused on classifying patients into graded risk groups rather than trying to predict actual survival times. Several methods based on Cox's proportional hazard model have been developed for survival risk modeling in the $p > n$ setting (where the number of candidate predictors p exceeds the number of cases n). For these models, the log hazard function at time t for an individual with covariate vector $\underline{x} = (x_1, x_2, \ldots x_p)$ is of the form $\log\left(h(t, \underline{x})\right) = \log(h_0(t)) + \underline{\beta}'\underline{x}$. The attraction of the proportional hazards model is that the regression coefficients β can be estimated without specification of the baseline hazard function $h_0(t)$. With the method of supervised principal components (Bair & Tibshirani, 2004, 191), the first q principal components of the variables with the strongest univariate correlation with survival are used as the predictors in the proportional hazards model. As alternatives to supervised principal components, several authors have used partial least squares projections as variables in the proportional hazards model (Li & Gui, 2004, 663; Nguyen & Rocke, 2002, 67; Park, Tian, & Kohane, 2002, 790) or compound covariates (Matsui et al. 2012). If principal components or some other dimension reduction projection is not used, then the regression coefficient vector is estimated by maximizing the log partial likelihood with a penalty on the number and size of the regression coefficients (Tibshirani, 1997, 788; vanHouwelingen et al., 2006, 660). The several approaches to survival risk prediction have been reviewed and compared by Bovelstad et al. (2007, 661) and vanWieringen et al. (2009, 792).

Survival modeling is usually performed to classify patients into two or more risk groups. The survival outcome for a group of patients is usually summarized by computing the Kaplan–Meier estimate of the survival function for that group. The Kaplan–Meier estimates for the risk groups computed on the same set of data used to develop the survival model are, however, biased. Figure 2.1 shows results from a simulation performed by Subramanian and Simon (2010, 719) for high-dimensional survival modeling. There were 129 cases whose survival times and censoring indicators were known. Five thousand random variables were simulated from the standard normal distribution independently of the survival data. All 129 cases were used as training sets. A survival risk model involving feature selection and proportional hazards modeling was developed on the training set, and the same training set patients were then classified into high and low risk based on whether their predictive index was above or below the median. Kaplan–Meier survival estimates for these training set risk groups are shown in Figure 2.1 (left). Figure 2.1 (right) shows the Kaplan–Meier estimates for the risk classification of the corresponding classifiers on independent test set patients. The enormous bias of resubstitution estimates of the survival distributions of survival of the risk groups is apparent. None of the models is of any value for classifying future patients, although the resubstitution analysis of the training sets would misleadingly suggest otherwise.

B.6.2 Cross-Validated Kaplan–Meier Curves

Simon et al. (2011, 836) developed a cross-validation-based method for estimating the survival distribution of two or more survival risk groups for use when the number of cases is too small for effective sample splitting and this method is implemented in survival risk modeling tools in BRB-ArrayTools (Simon et al., 2007). To develop a cross-validated estimate of the survival distributions of the risk groups, the full data set D is partitioned into K approximately equal parts $D_1, \ldots, D_K$. One then starts with forming a training set $T_1 = D - D_1$ by omitting the first subset of cases D_1. A survival risk model M_1 is developed using *only* the data in T_1 for variable selection, regression coefficient fitting, and tuning parameter optimization. One can then classify each of the cases in the test set D_1 into a survival risk group. One specifies in advance how many risk groups are of interest and how patients will be classified based on the models developed. For example, one might classify patients as low risk if their predicted probability of surviving five years is at least 0.75, high risk if their predicted probability is less than 0.5, and intermediate risk otherwise. This is repeated for each of the K loops of the cross-validation. At the second step, another survival risk model is developed from scratch using training set $T_2 = D - D_2$. Both variable selection and model calibration are reperformed using only data in T_2.

After the cross-validation is complete, all cases have been classified into risk groups using a model developed on a training set of which they were not part. Kaplan–Meier curve estimates can be computed for each of the risk groups; that is, the patients classified as low risk over all loops of the cross-validation are grouped together, and a Kaplan–Meier estimator is computed.

For proportional hazards models, survival risk group assignment may be based on the cross-validated predictive index instead of the predicted probability of survival beyond t, thereby avoiding the need to estimate the cumulative baseline hazard in each training set T_k. For example, if two approximately equal risk groups are desired, a case i in partition D_k can be assigned to the higher risk group if its cross-validated predictive index $b^{(k)} x_i$ is below the median of the full set of all cross-validated predictive indices in T_k.

Figure B.2a shows the resubstitution estimate of Kaplan–Meier curves for the training set data reported by Shedden et al. (2008, 625). Figure B.2b shows the cross-validated Kaplan–Meier curves for those same data.

Although the log-rank statistic is a convenient measure of spread among the cross-validated survival curves, the log-rank test is not valid

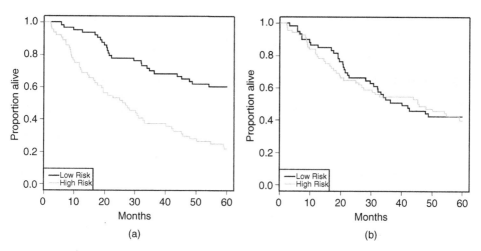

Figure B.2. (a) Resubstitution estimates of Kaplan–Meier curves for high-risk and low-risk prognostic groups when the same data are used for developing the prognostic model and for calculating the Kaplan–Meier curves. Data for the training set are data reported by Shedden et al. (2008, 625). (b) Cross-validated Kaplan–Meier curves for the same data.

because the curves are cross-validated survival curves, and hence the observations are not independent. To evaluate the statistical significance of the log-rank statistic, we obtain the permutation distribution of the cross-validated log-rank statistic; that is, we randomly permute the correspondence of survival times and censoring indicators to different gene expression profiles and repeat the entire K-fold cross-validation process. Then we compute the cross-validated survival curves and the cross-validated log-rank statistic for that random permutation. We repeat that entire process for many random permutations and generate the null distribution of the cross-validated log-rank statistic. The proportion of replicates with a log-rank statistic greater than or equal to the value of the statistic for the unpermuted data is the statistical significance level for the test that survival is independent of all covariates. For the cross-validated Kaplan–Meier curves shown in Figure B.2b, the log-rank statistic is 0.12, and the statistical significance level was 0.85 based on 500 random permutations. Survival risk modeling with cross-validated Kaplan-Meier curves and significance assessed by the permutation distribution of the log-rank statistic is provided in the BRB-ArrayTools software available at http://brb.nci.nih.gov (Simon et al., 2007, 2011, 836).

B.6.3 Time-Dependent Receiver Operating Characteristic Curves

For binary disease classification problems (i.e., disease vs. no disease), the commonly used measures of predictive accuracy are sensitivity, specificity, positive predictive value, negative predictive value, and receiver operating characteristic (ROC) curve (Pepe et al., 2004, 701). Suppose we have a quantitative test result M and that values greater than a threshold c are considered positive and predictive of disease presence ($D = 1$). The sensitivity and specificity of the test are defined as $\Pr[M \geq c \mid D = 1]$ and $\Pr[M < c \mid D = 0]$, respectively. An ideal test has sensitivity and specificity of 1. A plot of sensitivity versus $1 -$ specificity as the threshold c varies is called the ROC curve. If the test is uninformative, the plot will be the diagonal line $y = x$ and the area under the curve will be 0.5. The area under the ROC curve is frequently taken as a measure of predictive accuracy of the test. The positive and negative predictive values are defined as $\Pr[D = 1 \mid M \geq c]$ and $\Pr[D = 0 \mid M < c]$, respectively. They are important in practice but are less frequently used for evaluation of tests in developmental studies because they depend on the prevalence of the disease $\Pr[D = 1]$, which may vary among contexts of use of the test.

Heagerty, Lumley, and Pepe (2000, 681) defined measures of sensitivity, specificity, and ROC curve for use with survival data. These are based on a defined landmark time t. The sensitivity and specificity are defined as $\Pr[M \geq c \mid T \leq t]$ and $\Pr[M < c \mid T > t]$, respectively, where T is the random variable denoting survival time, M is the test value, and c is the threshold of positivity. Hence, survival less than landmark time t is taken to be the "disease" class. Subramanian and Simon (2011, 837) proposed that for applications with proportional hazards survival risk models, the test value M for a patient is taken as the cross-validated predictive index for that patient. Using Bayes's theorem, sensitivity and specificity can be estimated as

$$\Pr[M \geq c | T \leq t] = \Pr[T \leq t | M \geq c] \, \Pr[M \geq c] / \Pr[T \leq t] \quad (B.3)$$

and

$$Pr[M < c|T > t] = Pr[T > t|M < c] Pr[M < c] / Pr[T > t]. \quad (B.4)$$

Kaplan–Meier estimators of the terms $Pr[T \leq t \mid M \geq c]$ and $Pr[T > t \mid M < c]$ can be computed for subsets of patients with $M \geq c$ and $M < c$, respectively. The denominators in (B.3) and (B.4) can be estimated by Kaplan–Meier estimators for the entire set of cases. The term $Pr[M \geq c]$ is just the proportion of cases with cross-validated predictive indices greater than or equal to the threshold c. Heagerty et al. also provide nearest neighbor estimators of the sensitivity and specificity as functions of the threshold c that ensure monotonicity as a function of the landmark time. A plot of the sensitivity versus 1 – specificity for a fixed landmark time is called the time-dependent ROC curve. It can be estimated for various values of the landmark time t. The area under the time-dependent ROC curve (AUC) can be used as a measure of predictive accuracy for the survival risk group model. If the cross-validated predictive indices are used for the test values, then the time-dependent ROC curve is cross-validated. Subramanian and Simon (2011, 837) used this approach to evaluate different resampling procedures for estimating predictive accuracy of a variety of survival risk modeling approaches. Cross-validated time dependent ROC curves for high dimensional survival modeling is also provided in BRB-ArrayTools (Simon et al., 2007).

One can determine the null distribution of the area under the cross-validated time-dependent ROC curve by permuting the survival times (and censoring indicators), repeating the cross-validation procedure to create the cross-validated predictive indices for the permuted data, and recomputing the cross-validated time-dependent ROC curve and the area under the curve. This can be repeated for multiple permutations to generate the null distribution and the BRB-ArrayTools software provides this analysis. Figure B.3 shows the cross-validated time-dependent ROC curve for the Shedden et al. (2008, 625) data in Figure B.2. The area under this curve is 0.53, and the statistical significance level of the test that this AUC = 0.5 is 0.25 based on 500 random permutations.

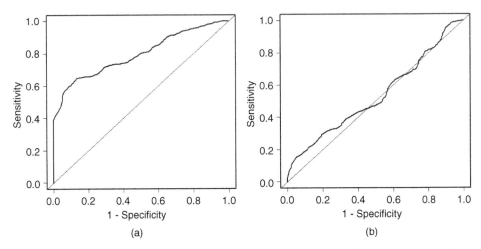

Figure B.3. The resubstitution estimate and the cross-validation estimate of the time-dependent ROC curve for the data of Shedden et al. (2008, 625).

B.7 Evaluating Whether a Prognostic Classifier Improves on Existing Prognostic Factors

Many disease areas utilize standard staging systems or standard clinical and histologic prognostic variables for evaluating patient prognoses. To have medical utility, a new prognostic classifier should provide classifications that are more refined than those provided using the accepted clinical or histopathological measurements (Kattan, 2003, 352; 2004, 353). The methods described above can be used to evaluate whether genomic variables add survival risk discrimination to a model based on standard covariates. Even prognostic models that provide more refined predictions than standard models will not necessarily find application, however. Medical tests are generally only ordered or reimbursed if they help with therapeutic decision making or other aspects of patient management. The analysis of the study should be focused on evaluating whether the new measurements provide an improvement over standard covariates for the intended use of the test, and the intended use should be the focus of the study.

Several approaches to developing combined survival risk models are possible. The BRB-ArrayTools software includes the supervised principal component approach (Simon, 2011, 836). For each training set, genes are selected for the combined model by fitting p proportional hazards regressions, each containing a single gene, and all the clinical covariates. Genes are selected if their expression adds significantly to the clinical covariates. The first few (q) principal components of those selected genes are computed for the training set, and a proportional hazards model is fit to the training set using those q principal components and the clinical covariates. That model is used to compute the predictive index for the test cases, and the test set cases are assigned to a risk group. When all K loops of the cross-validation are completed, the cross-validated Kaplan–Meier curves for the combined model are computed for these predicted risk groups.

Other methods of building combined models are also possible. For example, one can use L1 penalized proportional hazards regression, in which the penalty applies only to the gene expression variables and the clinical covariates are automatically included in the model. Whatever method is used for building combined models containing the standard covariates and the gene expression measurements, one uses the approach described earlier to obtain cross-validated predictive indices for the combined model. One can compute cross-validated Kaplan–Meier curves for the combined model based on grouping cases into risk groups based on these cross-validated predictive indices. One can similarly obtain cross-validated predictive indices for the standard covariate-only model. With very few standard covariates and many cases, it may not be necessary to cross-validate the model containing all the standard covariates. It is best to cross-validate the standard covariate-only models, however, because overfitting can become a problem even for models when the number of variables is much less than the number of cases or events.

We can compare the combined survival risk model to the model based only on standard covariates using as a test statistic the cross-validated log-rank statistic for the combined model minus the log-rank statistic for cross-validated Kaplan–Meier curves for the standard covariate model. The difference in areas under the cross-validated time-dependent ROCs curves can be used as an alternative test statistic. The null distribution of the test statistic is generated by permuting the gene expression vectors among cases. In these permutations, the correspondence between survival time, censoring indicator, and standard covariates is not disrupted. Evaluating the predictive discrimination of the new classifier within the risk groups defined by the standard classification is the most informative way to present the results (Cook, 2007).

References

Allegra C, Jessup JM, Somerfield MR, et al. American Society of Clinical Oncology provisional clinical opinion: Testing for KRAS gene mutations in patients with metastatic colorectal carcinoma to predict response to anti-epidermal growth factor receptor monoclonal antibody therapy. *Journal of Clinical Oncology.* 2009;epub JCO.2009.21.9170.

Amado RG, Wolf M, Peeters M, et al. Wild-type KRAS is required for panitumumab efficacy in patients with metastatic colorectal cancer. *Journal of Clinical Oncology.* 2008;26(10):1626–1634.

Bair E, Tibshirani R. Semi-supervised methods to predict patient survival from gene expression data. *PLoS Biology.* 2004;2:511–522.

Beckman RA, Clark J, Chen C. Integrating predictive biomarkers and classifiers into oncology clinical development programs. *Nature Reviews Drug Discovery.* 2011;10:735–748.

Ben-Dor A, Bruhn L, Friedman N, Nachman I, Schummer M, Yakhini Z. Tissue classification with gene expression profiles. *Journal of Computational Biology.* 2000;7:559–584.

Berger JO. *Statistical Decision Theory and Bayesian Analysis.* New York: Springer; 2010.

Bo TH, Jonassen I. New feature subset selection procedures for classification of expression profiles. *Genome Biology.* 2002;3(4):0017.1–0017.11.

Bogaerts J, Cardoso F, Buyse M, et al. Gene signature evaluation as a prognostic tool: challenges in the design of the MINDACT trial. *Nature Clinical Practice: Oncology.* 2006;3(10):540–551.

Bovelstad HM, Nygard S, Storvold HL, et al. Predicting survival from microarray data – a comparative study. *Bioinformatics.* 2007;23 (16):2080–2087.

Cai T, Tian L, Wong PH, Wei LJ. Analysis of randomized comparative clinical trial data for personalized treatment selections. *Biostatistics*. 2011;12:270–282.

Cook NR. Use and misuse of the receiver operating characteristic curve in risk prediction. *Circulation*. 2007;115(7):928–935.

Cox DR. Regression models and life-tables. *Journal of the Royal Statistical Society B*. 1972;34:187–220.

Cox DR, Snell EJ. *Analysis of Binary Data*. Boca Raton FL, Chapman and Hall/CRC; 1989.

Cronin M, Sangli C, Liu M-L, et al. Analytical validation of the Oncotype DX genomic diagnostic test for recurrence prognosis and therapeutic response prediction in node-negative, estrogen receptor-positive breast cancer. *Clinical Chemistry*. 2007;53(6):1084–1091.

Crowley J, Hoering A eds. *Handbook of Statistics in Clinical Oncology*, 3rd ed. Boca Raton, FL: Chapman Hall/CRC; 2012.

Deutsch JM. Evolutionary algorithms for finding optimal gene sets in microarray prediction. *Bioinformatics*. 2003;19:45–54.

Dobbin K, Simon R. Sample size determination in microarray experiments for class comparison and prognostic classification. *Biostatistics*. 2005;6:27–38.

Dobbin K, Simon R. Sample size planning for developing classifiers using high dimensional DNA expression data. *Biostatistics*. 2007;8:101–117.

Dobbin K, Simon R. Optimally splitting cases for training and testing high dimensional classifiers. *BMC Medical Genomics*. 2011;4:31.

Dobbin KK, Zhao Y, Simon RM. How large a training set is needed to develop a classifier for microarray data? *Clinical Cancer Research*. 2008;14:108–114.

Dudoit S, Fridlyand J. Classification in microarray experiments. In: Speed T, ed. *Statistical Analysis of Gene Expression Microarray Data*. Boca Raton, FL: Chapman and Hall/CRC; 2003:93–158.

Dudoit S, Fridlyand J, Speed TP. Comparison of discrimination methods for the classification of tumors using gene expression data. *Journal of the American Statistical Association*. 2002;97:77–87.

Dupuy A, Simon R. Critical review of published microarray studies for cancer outcome and guidelines on statistical analysis and reporting. *Journal of the National Cancer Institute*. 2007;99:147–157.

Ellenberg S, Fleming TR, DeMets D. *Data Monitoring Committees in Clinical Trials: A Practical Perspective.* New York: Wiley; 2002.

Fisher RA. The use of multiple measurements in taxonomic problems. *Annals of Eugenics.* 1936;7:179–188.

Fleming TR. Interpretation of subgroup analyses in clinical trials. *Drug Information Journal.* 1995;29:1681S–1687S.

Fleming TR, Watelet L. Approaches to monitoring clinical trials. *Journal of the National Cancer Institute.* 1989;188–193.

Foster JC, Taylor JMG, Ruberg SJ. Subgroup identification from randomized clinical trial data. *Statistics in Medicine.* 2011;30:2867–2880.

Fox E, Curt GA, Balis FM. Clinical trial design for target-based therapy. *The Oncologist* 2002;7:401–409.

Freidlin B, Jiang W, Simon R. The cross-validated adaptive signature design for predictive analysis of clinical trials. *Clinical Cancer Research.* 2010;16(2):691–698.

Freidlin B, McShane LM, Korn EL. Randomized clinical trials with biomarkers: design issues. *Journal of the National Cancer Institute.* 2010;102(3):152–160.

Freidlin B, Simon R. Adaptive signature design: an adaptive clinical trial design for generating and prospectively testing a gene expression signature for sensitive patients. *Clinical Cancer Research.* 2005;11:7872–7878.

Freidlin B, McShane LM, Polley MY, Korn EL. Randomized phase II trial designs with biomarkers. *Journal of Clinical Oncology.* 2012;30(30):3304–3309.

Golub TR, Slonim DK, Tamayo P, et al. Molecular classification of cancer: class discovery and class prediction by gene expression monitoring. *Science.* 1999;286:531–537.

Green S, Benedetti J, Crowley J. *Clinical Trials in Oncology.* 2nd ed. Boca Raton FL: Chapman and Hall/CRC; 2003.

Harrell FE. *Regression Modeling Strategies with Applications to Linear Models, Logistic Regression and Survival Analysis.* New York: Springer; 2001.

Hastie T, Tibshirani R, Eisen M, et al. Gene shaving as a method for identifying distinct sets of genes with similar expression patterns. *Genome Biology.* 2000;1(2)3.1–3.21.

Hastie T, Tibshirani R, Friedman J. *The Elements of Statistical Learning: Data Mining, Inference, and Prediction*, 2nd ed. New York: Springer; 2009.

Haybittle JL. Repeated assessment of results in clinical trials of cancer treatment. *Journal of Radiology*. 1971;44:793.

Hayes DF, Bast RC, Desch CE, et al. Tumor marker utility grading system: a framework to evaluate clinical utility of tumor markers. *Journal of the National Cancer Institute*. 1996;88:1456–1466.

Heagerty PJ, Lumley T, Pepe MS. Time dependent ROC curves for censored survival data and a diagnostic marker. *Biometrics*. 2000;56:337–344.

Hess KR, Anderson K, Symmans WF, et al. Pharmacogenomic predictor of sensitivity to preoperative paclitaxel and 5-flurouracil, doxorubicin, cyclophosphamide chemotherapy in breast cancer. *Journal of Clinical Oncology*. 2006;24(26):4236–4244.

Hoering A, LeBlanc M, Crowley JJ. Randomized phase III clinical trial designs for targeted agents. *Clinical Cancer Research*. 2008;14:4358–4367.

Hsieh FY, Lavori PW. Sample-size calculations for the Cox proportional hazards regression model with nonbinary covariates, *Controlled Clinical Trials*. 2000;21:552–560.

Hunsberger S, Zhao Y, Simon R. A comparison of phase II study strategies. *Clinical Cancer Research*. 2009;15(19):5950–5955.

Jennison C, Turnbull BW. *Group Sequential Methods with Applications to Clinical Trials*. Boca Raton, FL: Chapman and Hall; 1999.

Jiang W, Freidlin B, Simon R. Biomarker adaptive threshold design: a procedure for evaluating treatment with possible biomarker-defined subset effect. *Journal of the National Cancer Institute*. 2007;99:1036–1043.

Jones CL, Holmgren E. An adaptive Simon two-stage design for phase 2 studies of targeted therapies. *Contemporary Clinical Trials*. 2007;28:654–666.

Kalbfleisch JD, Prentice RL. *The Statistical Analysis of Failure Time Data*. New York: Wiley; 2002.

Kaplan EI, Meier P. Nonparametric estimation from incomplete observations. *Journal of the American Statistical Association*. 1958;53:457–481.

Karapetis CS, Khambata-Ford S, Jonker DJ, et al. K-ras mutations and benefit from cetuximab in advanced colorectal cancer. *New England Journal of Medicine.* 2008;359(17):1757–1765.

Karuri S, Simon R. A two-stage Bayesian design for co-development of new drugs and companion diagnostics. *Statistics in Medicine.* 2012; 31(10):901–914.

Kattan MW. Judging new markers by their ability to improve predictive accuracy. *Journal of the National Cancer Institute.* 2003;95(9):634–635.

Kattan MW. Evaluating a new marker's predictive contribution. *Clinical Cancer Research.* 2004;10:822–824.

Khan J, Wei JS, Ringner M, et al. Classification and diagnostic prediction of cancers using gene expression profiling and artificial neural networks. *Nature Medicine.* 2001;7:673–679.

Kim KI, Simon R. Probabilistic classifiers with high dimensional data. *Biostatistics.* 2011;12(3):399–412.

Korn EL, Freidlin B. Outcome-adaptive randomization: is it useful? *Journal of Clinical Oncology.* 2011;29:771–776.

Korn EL, Freidlin B, Abrams JS, Halabi S. Design issues in randomized phase II/III trials. *Journal of Clinical Oncology.* 2012;30(6):667–671.

Lai TL, Lavori PW, Shih M, Sikic BI. Clinical trial designs for testing biomarker-based personalized therapies. *Clinical Trials.* 2012;9:141–154.

Lai C, Reindders MJT, van't Veer LJ, Wessels LFA. A comparison of univariate and multivariate gene selection techniques for classification of cancer datasets. *BMC Bioinformatics.* 2006;7:235.

Lenz G, Wright GW, Dave SS, et al. Stromal gene signatures in large-B-cell lymphomas. *New England Journal of Medicine.* 2008;359(22):2313–2323.

Li H, Gui J. Partial Cox regression analysis for high-dimensional microarray gene expression data. *Bioinformatics.* 2004;20:i208–i215.

Liu A, Li Q, Yu KF, Yuan VW. A threshold sample-enrichment approach in a clinical trial with heterogeneous subpopulations. *Clinical Trials.* 2010;7(5):537–545.

Maitournam A, Simon R. On the efficiency of targeted clinical trials. *Statistics in Medicine.* 2005;24:329–339.

Mandrekar SJ, Sargent DJ. Clinical trial designs for predictive biomarker validation: Theoretical considerations and practical challenges. *Journal of Clinical Oncology.* 2009;27:4027–4034.

Mandrekar SJ, Sargent DJ. Predictive biomarker validation in practice: lessons from real trials. *Clinical Trials*. 2010;7:567–573.

Mantel N. Chi-square tests with one degree of freedom; extensions of the Mantel-Haenszel procedure. *Journal of American Statistical Association*. 1963;58:690–700.

Marubini E, Valsecchi MG. *Analysing Survival Data from Clinical Trials and Observational Studies*. New York: Wiley; 1995.

Matsui S, Simon R, Qu P, Shaughnessy JD, Barlogie B, Crowley JJ. Developing and validating continuous genomic signatures in randomized clinical trials for predictive medicine. *Clinical Cancer Research*. 2012; 18(21):6065–6073.

McShane LM, Hunsberger S, Adjei AA. Effective incorporation of biomarkers into phase II trials. *Clinical Cancer Research*. 2009;15(6):1898–1905.

Molinaro AM, Simon R, Pfeiffer RM. Prediction error estimation: a comparison of resampling methods. *Bioinformatics*. 2005;21(15):3301–3307.

Nguyen DV, Rocke DM. Partial least squares proportional hazard regression for application to DNA microarray survival data. *Bioinformatics*. 2002;18:1625–1632.

O'Brien PC, Fleming TR. A multiple testing procedure for clinical trials. *Biometrics*. 1979;35:549–556.

Ooi CH, Tan P. Genetic algorithms applied to multi-class prediction for the analysis of gene expression data. *Bioinformatics*. 2003;19:37–44.

Paik S, Shak S, Tang G, et al. A multigene assay to predict recurrence of tamoxifen-treated, node-negative breast cancer. *New England Journal of Medicine*. 2004;351:2817–2826.

Park PJ, Tian L, Kohane IS. Linking gene expression data with patient survival times using partial least squares. *Bioinformatics*. 2002;18:S120–S127.

Pepe MS. *The Statistical Evaluation of Medical Tests for Classification and Prediction*. New York: Oxford University Press; 2004.

Pepe MS, Janes H, Longton G, Leisenring W, Newcomb P. Limitations of the odds ratio in gauging the performance of a diagnostic, prognostic or screening marker. *American Journal of Epidemiology*. 2004;159:882–890.

Pepe MS, Feng Z, Janes H, Bossuyt PM, Potter JD. Pivotal evaluation of the accuracy of a biomarker used for classification or prediction: Standards for study design. *Journal of the National Cancer Institute.* 2008;100(20):1432–1438.

Peterson B, George SL. Sample size requirements and length of study for testing interaction in a $1 \times k$ factorial design when time-to-failure is the outcome. *Controlled Clinical Trials.* 1993;14:511–522.

Peto R, Pike MC, Armitage P. Design and analysis of randomized clinical trials requiring prolonged observation of each patient: II Analysis and examples. *British Journal of Cancer.* 1977;35:1–39.

Piantadosi S. *Clinical Trials: A Methodologic Perspective.* New York, Wiley; 2005.

Pocock SJ. Interim analyses for randomized clinical trials. *Biometrics.* 1982;39:153.

Pocock SJ, Assmann SE, Enos LE, Kasten LE. Subgroup analysis, covariate adjustment and baseline comparisons in clinical trial reporting: current practice and problems. *Statistics in Medicine.* 2002;21:2917–2930.

Pusztai L. Perspectives and challenges of clinical pharmacogenomics in cancer. *Pharmacogenomics.* 2004;5(5):451–454.

Pusztai L, Anderson K, Hess KR. Pharmacogenomic predictor discovery in phase II clinical trials for breast cancer. *Clinical Cancer Research.* 2007;13:6080–6086.

Radmacher MD, McShane LM, Simon R. A paradigm for class prediction using gene expression profiles. *Journal of Computational Biology.* 2002;9:505–512.

Rosenwald A, Wright G, Chan WC, et al. The use of molecular profiling to predict survival after chemotherapy for diffuse large-B-cell lymphoma. *New England Journal of Medicine.* 2002;346:1937–1947.

Rubin DB. *Bayesian Data Analysis.* Boca Raton FL, Chapman and Hall/CRC; 2009.

Rubin DB, van der Laan MJ. Statistical issues and limitations in personalized medicine research with clinical trials. *The International Journal of Biostatistics.* 2012;8:1–37.

Sargent DJ, Conley BA, Allegra C, Collette L. Clinical trial designs for predictive marker validation in cancer treatment trials. *Journal of Clinical Oncology.* 2005;23(9):2020–2027.

Sawyers CL. The cancer biomarker problem. *Nature*. 2008;452:548–552.

Shedden K, Taylor JMG, Enkemann SA, et al. Gene expression–based survival prediction in lung adenocarcinoma: a multi-site, blinded validation study. *Nature Medicine*. 2008;14(8):822–827.

Sher HI, Nasso SF, Rubin E, Simon R. Adaptive clinical trial designs for simultaneous testing of matched diagnostics and therapeutics. *Clinical Cancer Research*. 2011;17:6134–6140.

Simon R. Confidence intervals for reporting results from clinical trials. *Annals of Internal Medicine*. 1986;105:429–435.

Simon R. Optimal two-stage design for phase II clinical trials. *Controlled Clinical Trials*. 1989;10:1–10.

Simon RM, Korn EL, McShane LM, et al. *Design and Analysis of DNA Microarray Investigations*. New York: Springer; 2004.

Simon R, Lam A, Li MC, Ngan M, Menezes S, Zhao Y. Analysis of gene expression data using BRB-ArrayTools. *Cancer Informatics*. 2007;2:11–17.

Simon R. Using genomics in clinical trial design. *Clinical Cancer Research*. 2008b;14:5984–5993.

Simon R. Design and analysis of clinical trials. In: DeVita VT, DePinto RA, Lawrence TS, Rosenberg SA, Weinberg RA, eds. *Principles and Practice of Oncology*. 9th ed. Philadelphia: Lippincott, Williams, and Wilkins; 2011:Chapter 70.

Simon R. Clinical trials for predictive medicine. *Statistics in Medicine*. In press.

Simon R, Maitournam A. Evaluating the efficiency of targeted designs for randomized clinical trials. *Clinical Cancer Research*. 2005;10:6759–6763.

Simon R, Maitournam A. Evaluating the efficiency of targeted designs for randomized clinical trials: supplement and correction. *Clinical Cancer Research*. 2006;12:3229.

Simon RM, Paik S, Hayes DF. Use of archived specimens in evaluation of prognostic and predictive biomarkers. *Journal of the National Cancer Institute*. 2009;101(21):1–7.

Simon R, Radmacher MD, Dobbin K, McShane LM. Pitfalls in the use of DNA microarray data for diagnostic and prognostic classification. *Journal of the National Cancer Institute*. 2003;95:14–18.

Simon RM, Subramanian J, Li MC, Menezes S. Using cross validation to evaluate prediction accuracy of survival risk classifiers based on high dimensional data. *Briefings in Bioinformatics*. 2011;12(3):203–214.

Simon R, Wang SJ. Use of genomic signatures in therapeutics development. *The Pharmacogenomics Journal*. 2006;6:1667–1173.

Slamon DJ, Leyland-Jones B, Shak S, et al. Use of chemotherapy plus a monoclonal antibody against HER2 for metastatic breast cancer that overexpresses HER2. *New England Journal of Medicine*. 2001;344(11): 783–792.

Smith M, Ungerleider R, Korn E, Rubinstein L, Simon R. The role of independent data monitoring committees in randomized clinical trials sponsored by the National Cancer Institute. *Journal of Clinical Oncology*. 1997;15:2736–2743.

Song Y, Chi GYH. A method for testing a prespecified subgroup in clinical trials. *Statistics in Medicine*. 2007;26:3535–3549.

Sparano JA, Paik S. Development of the 21-gene assay and its application in clinical practice and clinical trials. *Journal of Clinical Oncology*. 2008;26(5):721–728.

Speed T, ed. *Statistical Analysis of Gene Expression Microarray Data*. Boca Raton, FL: Chapman and Hall/CRC; 2003.

Spiegelhalter DJ, Freedman LS, Parmar MKB. Bayesian approaches to randomized trials. *Journal of the Royal Statistical Society A*. 1994;157:357–387.

Subramanian J, Simon R. An evaluation of resampling methods for assessment of survival risk prediction in high dimensional settings. *Statistics in Medicine*. 2011;30(6):642–653.

Subramanian J, Simon R. Gene expression-based prognostic signatures in lung cancer: Ready for clinical use? *Journal of the National Cancer Institute*. 2010a;102:464–474.

Subramanian J, Simon R. What should physician look for in evaluating prognostic gene expression signatures. *Nature Reviews Clinical Oncology*. 2010b;7:327–334.

Taylor JMG, Ankerst DP, Andridge RR. Validation in biomarker based risk prediction models. *Clinical Cancer Research*. 2008;14:5977–5983.

Tibshirani R. The lasso method for variable selection in the Cox model. *Statistics in Medicine*. 1997;16:385–395.

Tibshirani R, Hastie T, Narasimhan B, et al. Diagnosis of multiple cancer types by shrunken centroids of gene expression. *Proceedings of the National Academy of Sciences of the United States of America.* 2002;99:6567–6572.

van-de-Vijver MJ, He YD, Veer LJvt, et al. A gene expression signature as a predictor of survival in breast cancer. *New England Journal of Medicine.* 2002;347(25):1999–2009.

vanHouwelingen HC, Bruinsma T, Hart AAM, van'tVeer LJ, Wessels LFA. Cross-validated Cox regression on microarray gene expression data. *Statistics in Medicine.* 2006;25:3201–3216.

van't-Veer LJ, Dai H, Vijver MJvd, et al. Gene expression profiling predicts clinical outcome of breast cancer. *Nature.* 2002;415:530–536.

vanWieringen WN, Kun D, Hampel R, Boulesteix AL. Survival prediction using gene expression data: a review and comparison. *Computational Statistics and Data Analysis.* 2009;53:1590–1603.

Varma S, Simon R. Bias in error estimation when using cross-validation for model selection. *BMC Bioinformatics.* 2006;7:91.

Wang SJ, O'Neill RT, Hung HMJ. Approaches to evaluation of treatment effect in randomized clinical trials with genomic subset. *Pharmaceutical Statistics.* 2007;6:227–244.

West M, Blanchette C, Dressman H. Predicting the clinical status of human breast cancer by using gene expression profiles. *Proceedings of the National Academy of Sciences of the United States of America.* 2001;98:11462–11467.

Zhang B, Tsiatis AA, Laber EB, Davidian M. A robust method for estimating optimal treatment regimens. *Biometrics* 2012 (Online May 2, 2012).

Zhao YD, Dmitrienko A, Tamura R. On optimal designs of clinical trials with a sensitive subgroup. *Statistics in Biopharmaceutical Research.* 2010;2(1):72–83.

Index

Note: An *f* following a page number refers to a figure on that page; a *t* following a page number refers to a table following that page.

adaptive
  eligibility, 55–57
  randomization, 31
adaptive signature design, 72–73, 74
  cross-validated, 75–79
  fall-back test, 47–48
adaptive threshold design, 59–63
  probabilistic indication classifier and, 60–62
  sample size planning, 62–63
aggregated Classification Trees, 117
algorithms
  class prediction, 112–118
  genetic, 114
  pre-specified algorithmic analysis plan, 72
analytical validity, 11, 88

baseline cumulative hazard, 122–123
baseline hazard function, 30, 120
Battle I trial in advanced non-small cell lung cancer, 30–33
  results of, 31*t*, 31–32
  two-stage design, 32–33
Bayesian methods, 101–103
  adaptive designs for randomized phase II trials, 30–33

computing posterior probabilities, 102–103
estimating sensitivity and specificity, 124
frequentist methods *versus*, 101–102
loss function, 102–103
non-informative prior distributions, 103
posterior distributions, 102
prior distributions, 102, 103
probabilistic indication classifier, 61
Type I error, 103
usefulness in phase 3 trials, 103
binary disease classification, 124–125
biomarkers. *See* predictive biomarkers; prognostic biomarkers
blinding
  assay to clinical data, 87, 88
  results of interim analyses, 5
bootstrapping, 61, 66, 79
BRB-ArrayTools software, 125
breast cancer
  enrichment design and trastuzumab, 39
  MammaPrint score, 11, 22, 33
  Oncotype DX recurrence score, 11, 22–23, 35
  TAILORx clinical trial, 22–23, 35, 86

calibration, 119–120

class comparison, 105–106, 107

class discovery, 105–106

class labels, 107–108, 109, 110, 111

class prediction, 105

    bias in estimate of error rates, 111

    components of, 107–108

    cross-validation, 68, 109–111

        leave-one-out-cross-validation, 109–111

    definition of, 107–108

    estimating accuracy of, 108–112

    feature selection, 108, 113–114

    mathematical classifier function, 108, 112–118

        classification trees, 117

        compound covariate, 70, 116

        Fisher discriminant analysis, 115, 116

        k-nearest neighbor, 117

        nearest centroid classification, 117

        nearest neighbor classification, 116, 117–118, 125

        support vector machines, 116

        weighted voting classifier, 69, 116

    misclassification rate, 116, 118

    parameter specification, 108

clinical trials. *See* phase 1 trials; phase 2 trials; phase 3 trials

clinical validity, 11, 85

cluster analysis, 106

companion diagnostic, 35–36, 88

Compound Covariate Predictor, 116

confidence interval, 66, 94–95

covariance matrix, 71, 99, 100, 119

Cox's proportional hazard model. *See* proportional hazards model

cross-validated Kaplan-Meier curves, 19*f*, 121–123, 127

cross-validation, 68, 109–111

adaptive signature design, 75–79

    error rate, 110–111

    leave-one-out-cross-validation, 109–111

    log-rank statistic, 128

    10-fold cross-validation, 78

data safety monitoring committee, 5

diagonal linear discriminant analysis, 115–116

enrichment design, 35–43

    sample size planning, 42–43

    standard design *versus*, 36–40

    test performance/specificity, influence on, 40

    trastuzumab study, 39

fall-back analysis, 47–48

false negatives

    in enrichment designs, 42

    in intention to treat analysis, 2

    in optimal two-stage design, 26

false positives

    in gene detection, 12–13

    in intention to treat analysis, 2

    in optimal two-stage design, 26

feature selection

    class prediction, 108, 113–114

    univariate gene selection, 79

Fisher linear discriminant analysis, 115

futility analysis, interim, 50, 56–57

gene finding, for prognostic classifier, 12–13

Gene Expression Omnibus, 78

gene expression profiles, to develop/validate prognostic classifiers, 105–128

gene shaving, 114

genetic algorithms, 114

genomics, vii, 46, 89

goodness of fit, 13–14

hazard function. *See* proportional
  hazards model

indication classifier, 46–47

intention to treat, 2

interaction design, 48

interaction tests, 48–49, 54

interim futility analysis, 50, 55–57

intermediate endpoint, 1, 25, 57

k-nearest neighbor classification, 117

Kaplan-Meier survival curves, 14–15, 16*f*,
    18, 96, 121, 125
  cross-validated Kaplan-Meier curves,
    19*f*, 121–123, 127

KRAS mutation status, 35, 83, 88

L1 penalized proportional hazards
    regression, 127

labels, class, 107–108, 109, 110,
    111

leave-one-out-cross-validation
    (LOOCV), 109–111

likelihood
  full likelihood, 99
  maximum, 98, 99
  partial, 100

linear discriminant analysis, 115–116

linear regression, 97, 98

LOE (Level of Evidence) Scale, 83

log-rank test, 76–79
  cross-validated statistic, 128

logistic regression, 28–29, 99

MammaPrint score, 11, 22, 33

Mann Whitney test, 113

marker strategy design, 21*f*, 20–21

matrix, covariance, 71, 99, 100,
    119

maximum likelihood, 98, 99

medical utility, 11, 20, 85

microarray analysis, 78. *See also*
    prognostic classifiers, based on
    high dimensional data

MINDACT clinical trial, 22–23

misclassification rate, 116, 118

modified marker strategy design, 22*f*,
    21–22, 23

molecularly targeted drugs, 1

multicenter clinical trials, 5

nearest centroid classification, 117

nearest neighbor classification, 116,
    117–118, 125

nearest shrunken centroid classification,
    118–119

noise variables, 108

non-informative prior distributions,
    103

nonparametric tests, 93

Oncotype DX recurrence score, 11,
    22–23, 35

one-sided p-value, 3

optimal two-stage phase II design,
    32–33

over-fitting, 68

p-value, 3
  one-sided, 3
  two-sided, 3

partial least squares, 114, 120–121

partial likelihood, 100

penalized logistic regression models, 72,
    119

permutation test, 65–67, 91–93

phase 2 trials, 25–33
    Battle I trial in advanced non-small cell
        lung cancer, 30–33
    Bayesian adaptive designs for
        randomized phase 2 trials, 30–33
    endpoint as progression-free survival,
        30
    logistic regression analysis, multiple
        candidate biomarkers, 28–29
    predictive biomarker design, single
        candidate binary, 26–28
    predictive biomarkers design, one or
        more binary candidates, 26
    purpose of, 1, 25–26
    two-stage design, 26
phase 3 trials
    endpoint, 2
    intention to treat principle, 2
    interim analyses, 4–5
    overview of, 1–5
    pivotal, 36
    power, 3–4
    purpose of, 45
    sample size, 3–4
    statistical significance of, 3
    subset analyses, 5
population sampling model, 93–94
pre-specified algorithmic analysis plan,
    72
predictive biomarkers
    designs based on single candidate
        biomarkers, 65–68
    designs for development/validation of
        multivariate classifiers, 68–79
    identification and validation of, 35–36
    logistic regression model, 28–29
    molecularly targeted therapy, 25, 53
    multiple, 65–79
    one or more binary candidates, 26
    predictive classifiers, 68

single candidate, 26–28
and study size, 4
predictive classifiers
    defining, 35
    development of, 106–107
    fall-back analysis and, 47–48
    indication classifier, 46–48
    randomized trial comparing new drug
        to control regimen, 36
    test performance/specificity, influence
        on enrichment design, 40
predictive pre-specified binary classifier,
        test positive/test negative patients,
        45–57
    adaptively modifying types of patients
        accrued, 55–57
    interaction tests, 48–49
    probabilistic indication classifier,
        49–52
    sample size planning, 52–55
probabilistic indication classifier, 49–52
    adaptive threshold design and, 60
    evaluation of sensitivity/specificity of
        classifier, 52
probability of early termination (PET),
        32t, 33t
probabilistic class prediction, 118–120
    refinement, 119–120
prognostic biomarkers
    classification error, 13
    false discoveries, 12–13
    goodness of fit and, 13–14
    medical utility of, 11
    sample size, 13
    split-sample approach to avoid bias,
        14–15. *See also* prognostic
        classifiers
prognostic classifiers
    based on high dimensional data,
        105–128

combined models, 127–128

evaluating whether, improves on existing prognostic factors, 126–128

marker strategy design, 20–21, 21*f*

medical utility of, 20

modified marker strategy design, 22*f*, 21–22, 23

univariate gene selection, 79

validation studies of, 20–23

prognostic factor studies, 11

proportional hazards model, 96–97, 99–101, 120

baseline cumulative hazard, 122–123

baseline hazard function, 30, 120

endpoint as progression-free survival, 30

hazard function, 96, 100

hazard ratio, 15

L1 penalized proportional hazards regression, 127

sample size planning, 4

prospective-retrospective design, 83–85

randomization

adaptive, 31

Bayesian designs and, 30–33, 49–50

stratified, 30, 45

re-sampling, 14, 125

re-substitution estimate, 111–112

of error rate, 111–112

regression modeling, 11, 97

linear regression, 97, 98

logistic regression, 28–29, 99

proportional hazards regression, 99–101

right-censored data. *See* survival data

ROC (receiver operating characteristic) curve, 124–125

cross-validated ROC, 125

sample size planning, 12–13, 52–55

and adaptive randomization, 31

adaptive threshold design, 62–63

enrichment design, 42–43

optimal two-stage design, 32–33

proportional hazards model, 4

sample splitting, 68

shrunken centroid classification, 117

split-sample method, 109

statistical power, 3–4, 96

statistical significance, 91–94

one-sided p-value, 3

permutation significance test, 65–67

threshold significance level, 4–5, 12, 113

two-sided p-value, 3

stratification design, 45

strong null hypothesis, 59–60, 76

study-wise type I error, 48–49

supervised principle component classifier, 114

support vector machines (SVMs), 116

survival analysis, 96–97

survival risk prediction, 120–125

cross-validated Kaplan-Meier curves, 19*f*, 121–123, 127

Kaplan-Meier survival curves, 14–15, 16*f*, 18, 96

survival risk classifiers, 120–121

time-dependent receiver operating characteristic curves, 124–125

t-test, 113

TAILORx clinical trial, 22–23, 35, 86

threshold significance level, 4–5, 12, 113

time-dependent receiver operating characteristic curves, 124–125

time-to-event endpoint, 54–55, 76–79

tuning parameters, 108

two-way analysis of variance, 48

type I error, 5, 83
   in adaptive signature design, 73
   and Bayesian methods, 103
   defined, 4–5
   study-wise, 48–49
   two-sided, 12
   without specifying cut-point in
      advance, 60

validity
   analytical, 11, 88
   calibration as measure of, 119–120
   clinical, 11, 85
   medical utility, 11, 20, 85
   of regression model, 101
   validation studies of prognostic
      classifiers, 20–23

Printed in the United States
By Bookmasters